LOWER YOUR
Blood
Pressure

Asparagus and
Wild Garlic Risotto,
page 82

LOWER YOUR
Blood
Pressure

A **21 DAY** DASH Diet Meal
Plan to Decrease Blood
Pressure Naturally

JENNIFER KOSLO,
PhD, RD, CSSD

ROCKRIDGE
PRESS

For general information on our other products and services or to obtain technical support, please contact our Customer Care Department within the U.S. at (866) 744-2665, or outside the U.S. at (510) 253-0500.

Rockridge Press publishes its books in a variety of electronic and print formats. Some content that appears in print may not be available in electronic books, and vice versa.

Photography © Gareth Morgans/Stockfood, cover; Reinhold Leitner/Shutterstock.com, cover; Bigacis/Shutterstock.com, cover; Clive Streeter/Stockfood, p. ii; Alex Luck/Stockfood, p. vi; Gräfe & Unzer Verlag/Anke Schütz/Stockfood, p. viii; Simon Desrochers/Stocksy, p. 2; Jill Chen/Stocksy, p. 18; Duet Postscriptum/Stocksy, p. 30; Gräfe & Unzer Verlag/Kramp + Gölling/Stockfood, p. 46 & back cover; Gräfe & Unzer Verlag/Thorsten Suedfels, p. 60; Trent Lanz/Stocksy, p. 86; Ivan Solis/Stocksy, p. 106 & back cover; Sara Remington/Stocksy, p. 128 & back cover; Susan Brooks-Dammann/Stocksy, p. 146; Natasa Mandic/Stocksy, p. 156.

TRADEMARKS: Rockridge Press and the Rockridge Press logo are trademarks or registered trademarks of Callisto Media Inc. and/or its affiliates, in the United States and other countries, and may not be used without written permission. All other trademarks are the property of their respective owners. Rockridge Press is not associated with any product or vendor mentioned in this book.

ISBN: Print 978-1-93975-422-6 | eBook 978-1-93975-423-3

This book is dedicated to my dad and brother and my other family members with high blood pressure, and to my mom for her undying support.

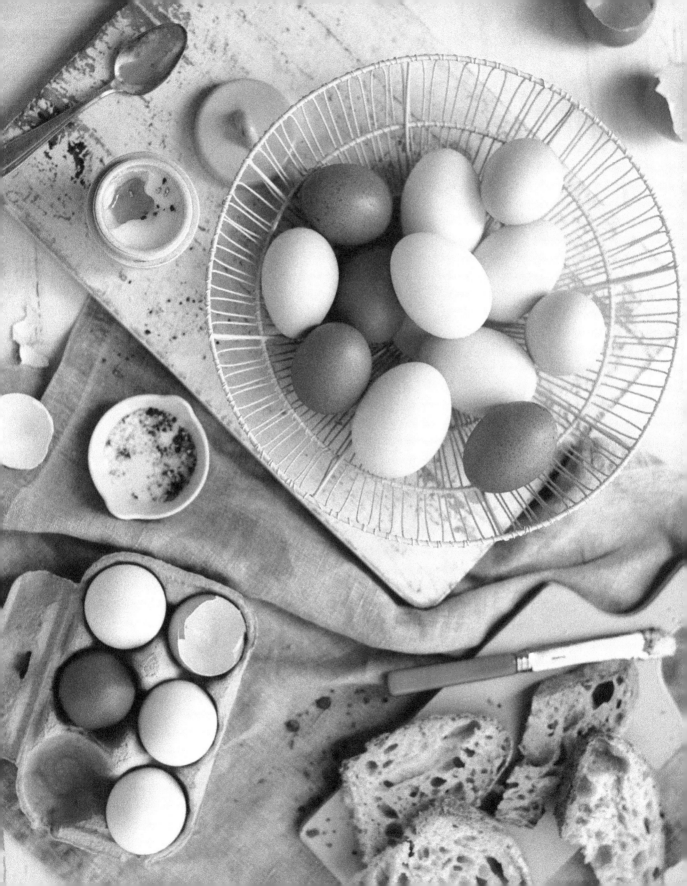

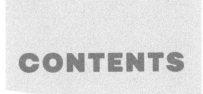

CONTENTS

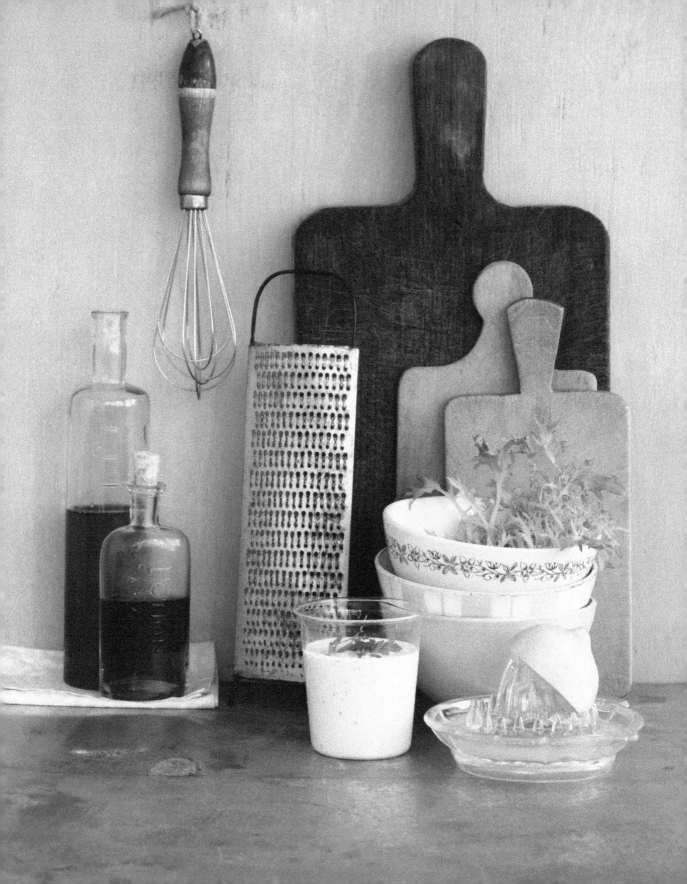

INTRODUCTION

I t can be frightening to hear those unfortunate words from your doctor—*You have high blood pressure*—and learn that uncontrolled high blood pressure (also known as hypertension) can lead to serious secondary issues such as strokes and heart attacks. If you or someone you love has been given this news, it can be a lot to take in. You likely have questions, including: "How long does it take to lower blood pressure?" and "What's the best way to do it?" The good news is that hypertension can usually be controlled through diet and lifestyle changes, and you may not need medication. Committing to dietary changes is by far the safer alternative. And, as you will learn in this book, changing your eating patterns doesn't have to be daunting.

As a registered dietitian nutritionist (RDN), I counsel many clients on how best to address high blood pressure. It's a disease that affects me personally, too. My father has high blood pressure, which he controls through a combination of dietary changes as well as medication. Since his diagnosis, my parents have made a 180-degree turn-about from the diet they were raised on to the way they eat now.

Both of my parents came from large families (and my dad was raised during the Great Depression) so my grandparents made food to feed a crowd: chipped beef, scrapple, sausage, and corn pies for my mom, who is of Irish and German descent; and lots of pierogis, lard and onion sandwiches, and kielbasa for my dad, who is Ukrainian. With such large families, my grandparents probably didn't have the time to worry about which foods offered the best nutrition. According to my mom, her mother certainly didn't, and neither did she as a young mother. When I was a child, feeding me was no picnic for my mom. I was a picky eater and had a natural dislike for some of the less-than-healthy traditional foods my mom prepared.

My career choice has allowed me to help my mother completely change her style of cooking over the years so that both she and my dad eat a healthy diet. These days, my mom makes nutrient-rich smoothies with lots of vegetables and fruits, prepares red meat only occasionally, and serves much more fish and poultry, more whole grains, lots of salads, and plenty of bean-based soups using lentils and black beans. My dad has given up soda and *never* puts salt on his food. And while my dad still needs medication to keep his blood pressure under control, he is in much better health today than he was years ago.

If you are new to the ways of healthy eating and my parents' story sounds familiar to you, I hope this book makes it easy for you to take preventative measures to help your hypertension and help you get started on the path to good nutrition and lower blood pressure. Food is powerful medicine, and eating well can improve your health.

The DASH diet is possibly the most-studied eating plan in history. (DASH is an acronym for Dietary Approaches to Stop Hypertension.) Numerous clinical trials have confirmed the effectiveness of DASH in lowering systolic blood pressure (the "top" number in a blood pressure reading) by as much as 11 to 14 points. This eating plan emphasizes more servings of fiber-rich carbohydrates (including whole grains, vegetables, and fruits), fewer servings of protein in general, and limited servings of red meat and sweets, along with boosting intake of low-fat dairy products and nuts and seeds.

By addressing issues with diet, you may be able to reduce your blood pressure without resorting to drug treatment. However, it is important to understand that there is a spectrum of healthy choices, and for some people, small changes are enough. If small or moderate changes don't work for you, it may mean you need to make bigger changes. Ultimately, we each need to personalize a way of eating and living that is right for us based on our needs, genes, and preferences. DASH is an excellent place to begin.

At this point in your journey, you may have all the technical information about hypertension, and you're now wondering *how* you can best address the issue. With that in mind, this book isn't meant to be an all-inclusive guide to managing hypertension. Instead, we'll focus on lifestyle changes that can help you lower your blood pressure naturally. Chapters 1 and 2 guide you step-by-step through lifestyle-change recommendations to help you ease into a new pattern of cooking, eating, and being active, and chapter 3 provides you with a 21-Day DASH-style meal plan, complete with shopping lists, so you can get started on making changes right away. Chapters 4 through 9 offer a variety of tasty recipes for every palate and preference.

I am grateful you have chosen this book. Before you know it, you will have created an eating plan you love!

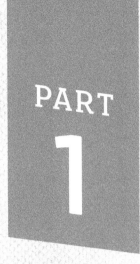

The DASH Lifestyle

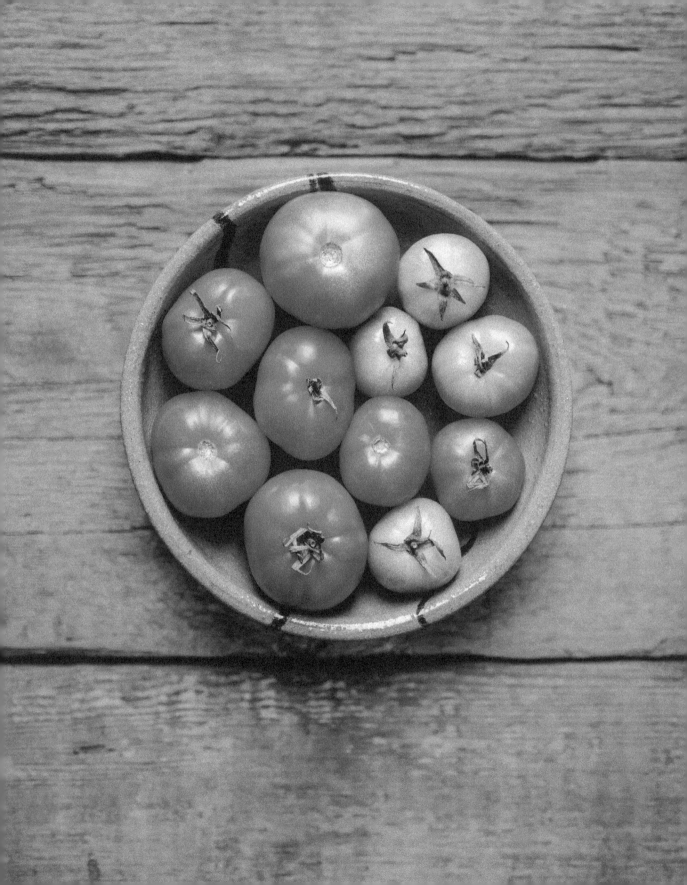

Starting Fresh

Controlling hypertension has become a national priority in the United States as part of the Million Hearts initiative from the Department of Health and Human Services, which aims to prevent 1 million heart attacks and strokes in the United States by the end of 2017 (for details on this initiative, check out MillionHearts.hhs.gov). Meanwhile, this chapter offers some basic information about hypertension, commonly called high blood pressure. If you are already familiar with the basics, feel free to jump ahead to chapter 2 or chapter 3. However, even if you are well-versed on the topic, this chapter can serve as a good refresher. You may even glean several new tips or pieces of information you were not previously aware of. If you are interested in additional information on hypertension, be sure to flip to the Resources section on page 163.

High Blood Pressure Basics

Blood pressure is the force of blood pushing against the walls of the arteries that carry blood from your heart to other parts of your body with each heartbeat. The magnitude of this force depends on how healthy your heart is and the amount of resistance of the blood vessels. The more blood your heart pumps and the narrower your arteries, the higher your blood pressure. While blood pressure normally rises and falls throughout the day, it can damage your heart and cause health problems if it stays high for a long time.

Hypertension, or high blood pressure, is the persistent increase in blood pressure above normal values. It is a common condition that, if left untreated, contributes to hardening of the arteries (atherosclerosis), stroke, heart attack, kidney disease or failure, vision loss, sexual dysfunction, angina (chest pain), peripheral artery disease (PAD), and the development of heart failure.

While the exact causes of high blood pressure are not known, there are a number of risk factors and conditions that play a role in its development. Some of those factors, called modifiable risk factors, are within your control, while others, called non-modifiable, are not. The following is a brief summary of the major risk factors.

Modifiable Risk Factors

Lifestyle: Greater intake of dietary salt (sodium), drinking too much alcohol (more than two drinks per day for men and more than one drink per day for women), too little potassium and calcium in the diet, too little vitamin D in the diet, using tobacco, and not being physically active.

Body weight: Being overweight or obese means more blood is needed to supply oxygen and nutrients to the tissues. As the volume of blood circulating through the blood vessels increases, so does the pressure on the artery walls.

Stress: Emotional stress, which causes a release of the stress hormones cortisol and adrenaline, can cause your arteries to constrict and your blood pressure to rise as part of the "fight or flight" response. Too much stress can also contribute to behaviors that increase blood pressure, such as poor diet, physical inactivity, and using tobacco or drinking excessive amounts of alcohol.

Non-modifiable Risk Factors

Age: Blood pressure rises naturally as we age, so the older we are, the more likely we are to get high blood pressure. However, children can also develop high blood pressure, a recent phenomenon attributed to the rise in overweight and obese children, and lack of physical activity.

BLOOD PRESSURE AND ETHNICITY

According to the Centers for Disease Control and Prevention (CDC), the prevalence of high blood pressure in African-Americans in the United States is among the highest in the world. More than 40 percent of non-Hispanic African-American men and women have high blood pressure, and it also develops earlier in life and is usually more severe. The problem is not limited to just adults. African-American preteens who are overweight may also develop high blood pressure.

Theories for why so many African-Americans have high blood pressure include higher rates of obesity and diabetes. Researchers have also found there may be a gene that makes African-Americans much more salt-sensitive. According to the American Heart Association, in people who have this gene, as little as 1 extra gram (half a teaspoon) of salt could raise blood pressure by as much as 5 mm Hg. Experts are also now looking into how socioeconomic disadvantages and lifestyle factors, such as less access to healthcare, lower levels of education and income, smoking, a poor diet, and a stressful lifestyle, may add to these risk factors. If you are an African-American with hypertension, work with your healthcare provider for the treatment plan and lifestyle changes that are right for you.

Gender: Until age 45, men are more likely to develop high blood pressure than women. From age 45 to 64, men and women develop high blood pressure at similar rates. At age 65 and older, women are more likely to develop high blood pressure than men.

Race: High blood pressure is more common in African-Americans, often developing at an earlier age and with more serious complications such as stroke, heart attack, and kidney failure. (See the sidebar on the previous page.)

Family history: High blood pressure has a genetic component and tends to run in families.

Blood Pressure Readings

The best way to know if you have high blood pressure is to have it checked. It is also important to understand what the numbers mean. Blood pressure readings have two numbers, usually written as 120/80 mm Hg (millimeters of mercury). The top number is called systolic pressure and the bottom number is called diastolic pressure. The ranges are:

- Normal: less than 120 over less than 80

- Prehypertension: 120-139 over 80-89

- Stage 1 high blood pressure (hypertension): 140-159 over 90-99

- Stage 2 high blood pressure (hypertension): 160 or higher over 100 or higher

- Hypertensive crisis (emergency care needed): 180 or higher over 110 or higher

- High blood pressure in people over age 60: 150 or higher over 90 or higher

Common Treatment Recommendations

While blood pressure naturally rises as we age and certain non-modifiable risk factors cannot be changed, there are steps you can take to keep your blood pressure within a normal range. These include: eating a healthy diet, getting regular exercise, reaching and maintaining a healthy weight, limiting alcohol, not smoking, and managing stress.

If you already have high blood pressure, you should get regular medical care and follow your prescribed treatment plan. Your plan will include healthy lifestyle recommendations and possibly medications. The following are the most common treatment recommendations.

Medication: High blood-pressure medications, known as antihypertensives, are available by prescription and include a variety of classes depending on your particular symptoms. More detail on medications is provided in the chart on page 8.

Diet: The DASH eating plan is the most recommended healthy-eating plan for controlling hypertension. Your physician will advise you on how strictly you will need to limit your sodium (salt) intake, and may also recommend that you limit your alcohol consumption.

Lifestyle: If you are overweight, your healthcare provider may suggest weight loss as well as a prescription of regular exercise. If you currently smoke, you will be asked to stop smoking. See chapter 2 for additional tips for incorporating regular physical activity into your routine.

By living a healthy lifestyle, you can help keep your blood pressure in a healthy range and lower your risk for heart disease and stroke. You have already taken the first step toward improving your health by choosing this book. Having high blood pressure is challenging, and you may think it is too hard to change your habits. However, small changes add up quickly over time and will have a lasting impact on your health.

MEDICATIONS COMMONLY USED TO TREAT HYPERTENSION

Although blood-pressure medications may have some troublesome side effects, many people find they are needed to keep blood-pressure readings within normal limits. Here's a quick rundown of the major classes of medications used to treat hypertension and their possible side effects. Your doctor will advise you whether or not medication is needed to control your hypertension. If you are currently taking medication, *do not* stop taking it, and never change your dose or your frequency without first consulting your doctor.

MEDICATIONS COMMONLY USED
TO TREAT HYPERTENSION

CLASS OF MEDICATION	HOW IT WORKS	COMMON SIDE EFFECTS
Diuretics (e.g., hydrochlorothiazide, chlorthalidone)	Diuretics help the body get rid of excess sodium and water to control blood pressure. They are often used in combination with other prescription therapies.	Some of these drugs may decrease your body's supply of potassium, resulting in weakness, tiredness, and leg cramps.
Beta-blockers (e.g., acebutolol, atenolol)	Beta-blockers reduce the heart rate, the heart's workload, and the heart's output of blood, which lowers blood pressure.	Possible side effects include insomnia, cold hands and feet, depression, and tiredness.
ACE (angiotensin-converting enzyme) inhibitors (e.g., lisinopril, benazepril)	ACE inhibitors help the body produce less angiotensin, which helps the blood vessels relax and open up, which in turn lowers blood pressure.	Possible side effects include skin rash, loss of taste, and dry hacking cough.
Angiotensin 2 receptor blockers (ARBs) (e.g., candesartan, losartan)	These drugs block angiotensin receptors so that the receptor fails to constrict blood vessels, which means the blood vessels stay open and blood pressure is reduced.	Possible side effects include dizziness.
Calcium channel blockers (e.g., amlodipine, diltiazem)	These drugs prevent calcium from entering the smooth muscle cells of the heart and arteries. By decreasing calcium, the heart's contraction is not as forceful. Calcium channel blockers relax and open up narrowed blood vessels, reduce heart rate, and lower blood pressure.	Possible side effects include palpitations, swollen ankles, constipation, headache, and dizziness. Grapefruit juice interacts with some calcium channel blockers, increasing blood levels of the medication and putting you at higher risk for side effects. Taking magnesium with these drugs may cause your blood pressure to drop too low.

CLASS OF MEDICATION	HOW IT WORKS	COMMON SIDE EFFECTS
Alpha blockers (e.g., doxazosin, prazosin)	These drugs reduce the arteries' resistance, relaxing the muscle tone of the vascular walls.	Possible side effects include fast heart rate, dizziness, and a drop in blood pressure upon standing.
Alpha-2 receptor agonists (e.g., methyldopa)	These drugs reduce blood pressure by decreasing the activity of the sympathetic portion of the involuntary nervous system.	Possible side effects include drowsiness and dizziness.
Combined alpha- and beta-blockers (e.g., carvedilol, labetalol hydrochloride)	Combined alpha- and beta-blockers are used as an IV drip for patients experiencing a hypertensive crisis. They may be prescribed for outpatient high-blood-pressure use if the patient is at risk for heart failure.	Possible side effects include a drop in blood pressure upon standing.
Central agonists (e.g., clonidine, guanfacine)	These drugs also help decrease blood vessels' ability to tense up or contract. The central agonists follow a different nerve pathway than the alpha- and beta-blockers, but also reduce blood pressure.	Possible side effects include a drop in blood pressure upon standing, drowsiness, dryness of the mouth, fever, and anemia.
Peripheral adrenergic inhibitors (e.g., guanadrel, reserpine)	These drugs reduce blood pressure by blocking neuro-transmitters in the brain. This blocks muscles from getting the signal to constrict. These drugs are rarely used unless other medications don't help.	Possible side effects include stuffy nose, diarrhea, and heartburn.
Vasodilators (e.g., hydralazine, minoxidil)	These drugs cause the muscles of the walls of the blood vessels to relax, allowing the vessels to dilate, which allows blood to flow through better.	Possible side effects include head-aches, swelling around the eyes, heart palpitations or aches, and pains in the joints.

The Dietary Difference

The DASH diet is specifically designed to help you lower your blood pressure by emphasizing foods rich in the minerals potassium, magnesium, and calcium—nutrients that promote a normal blood pressure. Named the best diet overall by *U.S. News & World Report* for the sixth year in a row as of 2017, DASH was developed in 1996 by researchers at several medical centers across the country. This diet is promoted by the National Heart, Lung, and Blood Institute (NHLBI), which is part of the National Institutes of Health.

The DASH eating plan is flexible, requiring no special foods, and instead focuses on daily and weekly nutritional goals. Depending on your individual calorie needs, there are several plans to choose from. The NHLBI website (www.nhlbi.nih.gov /health/health-topics/topics/dash/followdash) publishes a free guide that takes you through the process of determining your calorie requirements and how many servings of each food group you need. I will go into a little more detail later, but for now, here is a quick rundown of recommended daily servings for a 2,000-calorie diet:

- 2 to 2½ cups of fruits (equivalent to 4 to 5 servings)
- 2 to 2½ cups of vegetables (equivalent to 4 to 5 servings)
- 6 to 8 ounces of whole grains
- 6 ounces or less of meats, fish, and poultry
- 2 to 3 cups of nonfat or low-fat dairy foods
- 2 to 3 teaspoons of oil

In addition, DASH recommends four to five servings per week of nuts, seeds, and legumes. (A serving of nuts and seeds is 1 ounce; a serving of legumes is ½ cup.) DASH doesn't recommend cutting out sweets entirely, but suggests that dieters limit their intake to five servings per week. The DASH diet recommends no more than two alcoholic drinks per day for men, and no more than one for women.

There are two versions of DASH: On the standard DASH diet, you can consume up to 2,300 milligrams (mg) of sodium per day, and on the low-sodium DASH diet, the limit is 1,500 mg per day.

The NHLBI recommends you ease into the DASH diet, which you can do using the following guidelines.

Make sure you have plenty of color on your plate: Fruits and vegetables are naturally low in sodium and are rich sources of fiber, potassium, and magnesium. Aim to fill

50 percent of your plate at each meal with a variety of vegetables and fruits. Fresh, frozen, and canned all count—just choose canned without added salt.

Go for whole grain: Whole grains are high in cholesterol-lowering fiber, provide long-lasting energy, and are excellent sources of heart-healthy B vitamins and minerals. Choose brown rice, whole-wheat pasta, and whole-grain bread over their white counterparts.

Dine on dairy: Nonfat and low-fat dairy products are one of the best sources of calcium and vitamin D, two important nutrients for blood-pressure regulation. Dairy products also provide lean, high-quality protein. Choose low-fat yogurt and string cheese for snacks, cook soups with nonfat or low-fat milk, and choose nonfat or low-fat milk over soda for your drink.

Eat more plant-based meals: Beans and legumes are important sources of cholesterol and fat-free protein, fiber, minerals, and B vitamins. Consider instituting a meatless meal each week to boost your intake of plant-based foods.

Cook without salt and don't add salt to your foods at the table: When you start using the herbs and spices hiding in the back of your pantry, you won't miss the salt.

Buy fewer prepared and processed foods: These foods are generally high in salt. If you do buy prepared food, become label-savvy and aim for foods with 5 percent or less of the daily value of sodium.

Medication Warning: High blood pressure is a serious condition, so before making any drastic dietary or physical activity changes, consult with your physician and/or a qualified nutrition professional. Without your physician's approval, do not stop taking your medication under any circumstances. Remember, the content of this book is not intended to diagnose, treat, or cure your high blood pressure, so be sure to speak with your physician if you have any questions.

The recipes in this book are low in sodium and don't exceed the lower DASH limit of 1,500 mg of sodium per day. The ingredients have been chosen for their nutritional benefits, including those that are high in potassium, magnesium, calcium, fiber, and B vitamins, while being low in saturated and trans fat, cholesterol, and sodium. All fruits, vegetables, and grains in their natural forms are low in sodium, making it easy for you to plan your individualized DASH eating plan.

EATING ON THE DASH DIET

Choosing foods on the DASH diet is simple because this eating plan emphasizes the foods you have always been told to eat more of (fruit, veggies, whole grains, lean protein, and low-fat and nonfat dairy, beans, and nuts) and de-emphasizes the foods you have always been told to eat less of (fatty red meats, full-fat dairy products, sweets, sugar-sweetened beverages, and salt). An easy way to think about this is to fill 50 percent of your plate at breakfast, lunch, and dinner with fruits and veggies, 25 percent with whole grains, and 25 percent with lean protein, with two to three servings of fats and oils each day. You will also want to include two to three servings of nonfat or low-fat dairy products each day with meals or as snacks, and include four to five servings of nuts, seeds, and legumes each week. The following guidelines can help you plan your meals.

Foods to Enjoy Freely

Fruits: Aim for four to five servings per day and choose from all fruits, including those high in potassium such as bananas, apricots, and cantaloupe, as well as antioxidant-rich berries.

Vegetables: Aim for four to five servings per day and choose from all non-starchy vegetables, including summer squash, leafy greens, cruciferous veggies, tomatoes, and peppers.

Nonfat and low-fat (1%) dairy products: Aim to include two to three servings per day.

Beans and legumes: Aim to include four to five servings per week.

Foods to Enjoy in Moderation

Whole grains: Aim to fill 25 percent of your plate at each meal with whole grains, like whole-grain bread, brown rice, and whole-wheat pasta for a total of six to eight servings per day. Choose portions that match your energy expenditure.

Some fruits and vegetables: Avocados are high in healthy fats, but they are also calorie-dense, so keep an eye on portion sizes. Some vegetables are also very starchy and can be used in place of grains at meals, including sweet potatoes, potatoes (white, gold, and red), winter squash, corn, and peas. Each of these foods is a rich source of potassium, fiber, vitamins, and minerals, so do not omit them from your diet.

Reduced-fat dairy: Limit consumption of reduced-fat (2%) milk products to no more than one serving per day.

Nuts, nut butters, seeds: Aim for 1 ounce per day of nuts, or 2 tablespoons of nut butter, or ⅓ cup of seeds, or a total of four to five servings per week combined.

Lean meat, fish, and poultry: All fish, skinless white-meat chicken, skinless white-meat turkey, and lean cuts of red meat (including pork tenderloin, sirloin tip, top round roast, top sirloin, bison, and grass-fed beef) can be enjoyed up to 6 ounces per day depending on your individual calorie needs.

Foods to Eat Less Of

Refined grains: Limit consumption of pasta made with white flour, white breads, snacks made with refined flours, and white rice to no more than one serving per day.

Full-fat dairy products: Limit consumption of full-fat dairy products to no more than one serving per day.

Sweets: Keep intake of sweets to five or fewer servings per week.

Sugar-sweetened beverages: Reduce or eliminate consumption of soda and other sugar-sweetened beverages. (The American Heart Association recommends that women have no more than 100 calories or 6 teaspoons of added sugar per day; men 150 calories or 9 teaspoons per day.)

Processed foods: Frozen dinners, boxed rice and pasta mixes, most condiments, dressings, sauces, and seasoning mixes should be limited to as few servings as possible.

Salt: Limit sodium intake to a maximum of 2,300 mg per day or 1,500 mg per day, depending on your doctor's orders.

Foods to Avoid

Fatty red meat: Spare ribs, rib-eye, filet mignon, sausage, bacon, luncheon meats, hot dogs, smoked and cured meats, porterhouse, strip steak, and other very fatty cuts of pork and beef.

Saturated and trans fats: Avoid oils such as coconut oil and palm oil, processed snack foods, other trans-fat-containing foods, and other foods high in saturated fat.

Taking a natural approach to lowering your blood pressure is by far the safest and least expensive option. Medications are not only costly, but can come with some unwanted side effects. Unlike most other diets, DASH is not restrictive, offers variety, and is easy to follow as a lifelong dietary choice. DASH is a great option for anyone who wants to adopt a healthy diet.

Those Crucial Elements

When managing hypertension, two minerals in particular can be especially helpful. These include potassium and magnesium. Let's take a look at each.

Potassium

Potassium is a mineral found in most foods. In addition to helping your muscles contract and your nerves to function normally, it also helps balance fluids and minerals in your body. Most notably for our discussion, potassium also helps your body maintain normal blood pressure.

The recommended dietary allowance (RDA) for potassium varies depending on age. Children over age 13 and adults should get 4,700 milligrams (mg) of potassium per day, with the exception of lactating women, who require 5,100 mg per day.

Low potassium levels, or hypokalemia, can lead to weakness, lack of energy, high blood pressure, and other cardiac abnormalities. Common causes include inadequate dietary intake, improperly managed diabetes, excessive sweating, chronic alcoholism, diarrhea, and some heart medications. Abnormally high levels of potassium can lead to potassium toxicity, or hyperkalemia. Hyperkalemia most often affects individuals with chronic or acute kidney failure. Depending on your health conditions, you may need to increase or decrease your potassium intake—work with your healthcare provider to determine the amount right for you.

10 Foods High in Potassium:
1 medium banana (425 mg), 1 medium baked potato with skin (925 mg), 1 medium sweet potato with skin (450 mg), 1 medium tomato (290 mg), ½ cup of cooked pinto beans or lentils (400 mg), 3 ounces of baked or broiled salmon (319 mg), 6 ounces of yogurt (260 to 435 mg), 1 cup of nonfat, low-fat, or whole milk (350 to 380 mg), 1 cup of papaya (264 mg), and ½ cup of prune juice (370 mg).

COEXISTING CONDITIONS

When you have hypertension, your heart has to work harder and your risk for heart disease and kidney disease increases. Diabetes and hypertension often go hand in hand, most likely due to lifestyle factors. With some of these coexisting conditions, there are additional dietary concerns to be aware of. If you have a coexisting condition, work with your healthcare provider and a qualified nutrition professional before making any drastic changes to your diet.

Type 2 Diabetes: The DASH diet is one of the recommended eating patterns suggested by the American Diabetes Association for managing type 2 diabetes, in conjunction with regular exercise and maintaining a healthy weight (as noted by Alison Evert et al. in *Diabetes Care*). However, if you are taking medication to treat both type 2 diabetes and hypertension, it is important to be aware that some blood-pressure drugs may negatively affect your blood sugar and blood lipid levels. Find out from your doctor what your prescribed medicines might do.

Congestive Heart Failure: Most people who develop heart failure have (or had) another heart condition first. One of the most common conditions that can lead to congestive heart failure is high blood pressure. Making dietary changes can lessen the work the heart has to do, which can ease symptoms. It is recommended that people with heart failure keep sodium intake to less than 2,000 mg per day, and ideally 1,500 mg per day, as too much sodium causes the body to retain water, worsening the fluid build up that happens with heart failure.

Kidney Disease: The National Institute of Diabetes and Digestive and Kidney Diseases (NIDDK) recommends that people who have kidney disease work with a registered dietitian nutritionist for help following the DASH diet. In addition, a healthcare provider may suggest a diet that is also low in liquids to help reduce edema and lower blood pressure. It may also be recommended that people with kidney disease eat moderate or reduced amounts of protein, though the benefits of this are still being researched. Lastly, too much potassium may be harmful in people with kidney disorders because the kidneys become less able to remove it from the blood, causing it to build up to harmful levels.

Magnesium

Magnesium is an abundant mineral in the body, and it is naturally present in many foods. It is also a main ingredient in some over-the-counter medicines such as antacids and laxatives. The body requires magnesium for energy production, muscle and nerve function, blood-glucose control, and blood-pressure regulation, along with numerous other body processes.

The RDA for men ages 14 to 18 is 410 mg, ages 19 to 30 is 400 mg, and ages 31 to 50+ is 420 mg. The RDA for women ages 14 to 18 is 360 mg, ages 19 to 30 is 310 mg, and ages 31 to 50+ is 320 mg.

10 Foods High in Magnesium: 1 ounce of almonds (80 mg), ½ cup of cooked spinach (78 mg), 1 ounce of cashews (74 mg), ½ cup of cooked black beans (60 mg), ½ cup of cooked edamame (50 mg), 2 tablespoons of peanut butter (49 mg), 1 cup of cubed avocado (44 mg), 1 baked potato with skin (43 mg), ½ cup of cooked brown rice (42 mg), 1 cup of nonfat, low-fat, or whole milk (24 to 27 mg).

The National Institutes of Health reports that most older adults in the United States don't get the proper amount of magnesium in their diets, although extreme magnesium deficiency is rare. It's best to get the mineral from food, especially dark, leafy green vegetables, unrefined grains, and legumes. The American Heart Association does not currently recommend magnesium supplements for lowering blood pressure. Following a balanced, healthy diet will provide your body with the amount of magnesium you need. Work with your healthcare provider to determine if you need to make any dietary changes.

Making the Commitment

Adopting the DASH diet along with other healthy lifestyle changes is important for your long-term health and for reducing your blood pressure. However, you will experience a number of ups and downs in the short term and long term as your body adjusts to your new style of eating. The magnitude of these changes will be unique to you; we all have our own starting points in terms of health conditions, diet quality, and diet composition.

What to Expect in the Short Term

If you are currently following a more typical Standard American Diet (SAD), which tends to be high in processed and fast foods, refined carbohydrates, salt, and sugar, switching to the DASH diet may result in cravings for those foods as well as moodiness and maybe even headaches. It is important to ride out those cravings as they are only temporary. Once your body gets used to fresh, wholesome foods, your tastes will change and you will no longer crave less-healthy foods. On the positive side, you'll notice your hunger has stabilized, brain fog and low concentration is replaced by a higher level of clarity and focus, and you'll be amazed by how much food you can eat without gaining weight. You may even start to lose weight.

What to Expect in the Long Term

In the long term, you will find that you have much higher energy levels, you are losing weight, your digestion is more regular, and you are sleeping better. Depending on how closely you follow the DASH eating plan, you may be able to lower your blood-pressure readings by several points in just two weeks. Adopting the DASH diet will also lessen your risk for developing other chronic diseases, including type 2 diabetes, heart disease, certain cancers, and metabolic syndrome.

Set Realistic Goals

To keep motivation high, be certain to set realistic goals for yourself as you transition to the DASH diet. Reward, don't punish, and focus on each positive change you make rather than on the occasional slip-up. There are bound to be challenges along the way, so focus on the big picture and not the minutia—slow and steady wins the race. It takes time to learn new eating habits that will last the rest of your life.

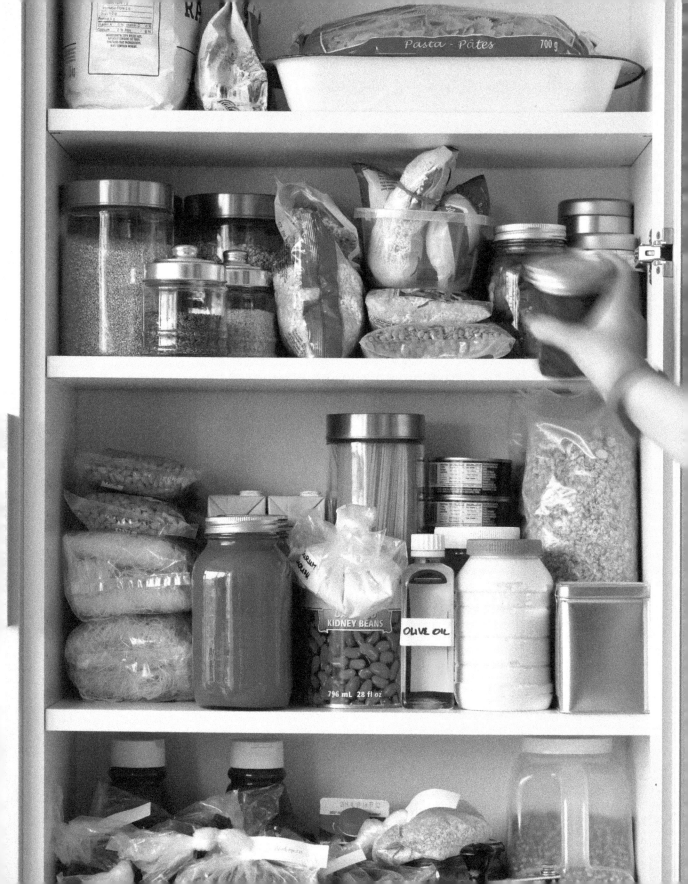

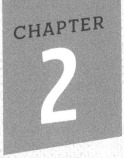

Going DASH, the Easy Way

Following the DASH eating plan is all about eating more whole foods and fewer processed foods, and achieving a certain number of daily servings from various food groups. There are no complicated rules to follow or strict food lists to adhere to. And while we all know that eating less sugar and salt and more fruits, vegetables, and whole grains will make us feel energized and healthier, beginning to make those changes can be daunting. Be patient with yourself along the way and remember that DASH is a healthy eating plan you can follow for life, so it's okay to transition slowly, making one change at a time. To help make your transition easier and more enjoyable, this chapter offers a step-by-step guide to get you started on your DASH eating plan.

Step 1: Clean It Out

Adopting the DASH eating plan is like embarking on a new lifestyle—a clean slate for you to make healthier food choices, lower your blood pressure, and more than likely drop a few pounds. To accommodate this new lifestyle, it is essential to set yourself up for success and make your environment foolproof so that when life gets busy and you're super hungry, your pantry and refrigerator will be filled with nutritious choices. A pantry clean-out is necessary to remove roadblocks to healthy eating and gets rid of those sugary, salty, and/or overly processed trigger foods. If an unhealthy food is in your possession, it's guaranteed that you or someone you love will eat it.

Before we get started, the first thing you need to do is to summon as much courage as possible. Purging will be painful, and you may experience feelings of anger and resentment. It feels wasteful to throw out perfectly good food. As you go through the following list, consider donating nonperishable items to your local food pantry. Perishable items can be given away, or you can simply toss them into your compost bin or trash if they're less than fresh. Grab some boxes and trash bags, and use this list to identify the foods in your pantry, refrigerator, and freezer that don't support your new lifestyle. All of the following need to go:

1. **Pre-prepared products:** While convenient, meals in a box such as macaroni and cheese, hamburger starters, and seasoned rice mixes all contain added sodium, preservatives, and added sugars. Canned soups are also extremely high in sodium.

2. **Sugary drinks, candy, snacks:** High in calories, sugar, additives, and sodium, foods like chips, cookies, sodas, most granola bars, and imitation juice drinks are devoid of nutrients and are simply empty calories.

3. **Certain condiments, salad dressings, and sauces:** Bottled seasonings are surprisingly high in sodium and added sugars, and contribute excess calories to your diet. In the case of salad dressings, they also contribute unhealthy fats.

4. **Refined breakfast cereals:** Read the nutrition facts panel of your cereal, and if it has less than 3 grams of fiber per serving, more than 200 mg of sodium per serving, and more than 6 grams of sugar per serving, donate it or toss it.

5. **Frozen foods:** Check your frozen fruits and vegetables, and if they contain added sauces, they will need to go. Frozen dinners are very high in sodium, added fats,

and sugars, and low in fiber, whole grains, and vegetables, making them poor choices.

6. **Refrigerated foods:** Luncheon meats, hot dogs, bacon, and sausage are notoriously high in sodium.

7. **Full-fat dairy products:** Opt for nonfat or low-fat dairy, and clear out the whole-fat sour cream, cream cheese, milk, and flavored yogurts.

Make healthier food options more visible or accessible. Environmental and visual cues strongly influence food intake. Place a bowl of fruit on your kitchen counter, keep washed and chopped vegetables eye-level in your refrigerator, and keep less-healthy options in a closed cabinet.

If you have housemates or family members who object to your pantry purge, you might first start by explaining that supporting you as you transition to the DASH eating plan will also improve their health. You might also strike a compromise and assign designated shelves in the pantry and refrigerator for family member treats. Because visual cues are so powerful, if you can have separate cupboards that would be even better—out of sight, out of mind.

Now that you have conquered your pantry purge, take a moment to pause and reflect on your progress so far in improving your health. Celebrating each success along the way will reinforce your resolve as you transform your eating plan.

Step 2: Stock Up

Now it's time for the fun part: restocking your pantry, freezer, and refrigerator with healthy, nutritious foods, and making the most of a tight budget without sacrificing flavor or variety. This section offers general guidelines for building a healthy pantry to get you ready for chapter 3, which provides shopping lists and pantry lists specific to the 21-day DASH meal plan.

If you can afford to purchase organic foods and free-range meats, that's great; it is always better to use cleaner ingredients. If buying all-organic would break the bank, check out appendix C (page 160). It contains the Environmental Working Group's annual list of the Dirty Dozen and Clean Fifteen, which you can use to review for foods you eat frequently, and, as budget allows, purchase only the Dirty Dozen foods organically. However, if you cannot afford organic foods at all, cooking with conventionally grown produce, canned produce, and conventional dairy and meats is still much healthier than eating processed and packaged foods.

In most cases, if you spend some additional time exploring your options at your local grocer, you will find that a number of low-sodium products exist and are readily available. Don't hesitate to speak to the store manager or department employees if you need help finding a certain food. The Resources section on page 163 provides a list of brands of reasonably priced healthy foods. Also, many of the recipes in part 2 include "Budget-Saver Tips" for cooking with frozen, dried, and canned ingredients.

The following list includes basic staples to keep on hand for preparing the recipes in this book, as well as meals that require little or no planning. Start with your budget in mind, and buy the staples you can afford. You don't need to purchase all of these ingredients before you start cooking, and this list is not exhaustive. Use the list for inspiration and build your healthy pantry over time until you have a well-stocked kitchen with healthy foods at your fingertips.

Pantry basics: Dry lentils; a variety of canned beans; canned no-salt tomatoes; low- and no-sodium vegetable and/or chicken broth; rolled oats; steel-cut oats; brown rice; whole-wheat pasta; unsalted nuts (almonds, pistachios); unsalted natural peanut butter; flavored vinegars; herbs and spices, including black pepper, basil, oregano, tarragon, thyme, dill, cumin, garlic, onion, and cinnamon; vanilla extract; cornstarch; whole-wheat flour; and unsweetened cocoa powder

Frozen vegetables: Spinach, broccoli, cauliflower, stir-fry vegetables, and peas

Fresh vegetables: Baby spinach or other leafy greens, broccoli, summer squash, mushrooms, tomatoes, onions, carrots, cabbage, and sweet potatoes

Frozen proteins: Skinless boneless chicken breasts, boneless fish fillets, shrimp, turkey breasts, and lean cuts of beef and pork

Fresh proteins: Eggs and tofu

Frozen fruit: Berries

Fresh fruit: Apples, bananas, citrus, lemon and lime juice; dried: apricots, and raisins

Dairy: Nonfat or low-fat milk (dairy or soy), nonfat or low-fat unflavored Greek yogurt, low-fat shredded cheese (including part-skim mozzarella), Parmesan cheese, and low-fat ricotta cheese

Fats and oils: Nonstick cooking spray, olive oil, and spreadable margarine

Step 3: Prepare Your Kitchen

Cooking is so much easier when you have the right tools on hand. Just like you did with your pantry, spend some time taking stock of your current tools, and organize your kitchen and workspace so your cooking can be effortless and your kitchen is a welcoming space. The recipes in part 2 require a minimal amount of equipment, but you will need some basics. Working within your budget, use the following two lists of "essential" equipment and "nice to have" equipment to choose your tools.

Essential Equipment

This list includes essential equipment for everyday cooking, aimed at the beginner cook.

Nonstick skillet/frying pan with lid: A good-quality nonstick skillet is an indispensable piece of equipment for browning, sautéing, and frying meats, fish, and vegetables. If you only purchase one size, choose a larger one, which will accommodate most recipes.

A large and small pot with lids: Pots will be used to prepare soups, sauces, and stews. Choose from glass, ceramic, stainless steel, and eco-friendly nonstick cookware. (Pots with nonstick coating require the use of less added fats and make for easy cleanup.)

Rimmed baking sheets: One or two 9-by-13-inch rimmed baking sheets are good to have on hand for roasting vegetables, meats, fish, and poultry. Metal is readily available, but you might consider silicone, which doesn't require greasing.

Assorted knives: Two types of knives are essential for cooking—a chef's knife for larger items like winter squashes and meats, and a small paring knife for fruits, vegetables, and herbs.

Cutting boards: Ideally you want two designated cutting boards—one for meats and one for fruits and vegetables, to limit the possibility of cross-contamination. If this isn't in your budget right now, choose one good-quality board, preferably made of wood, which is easy on kitchen knives. Always sanitize your board after working with raw meats and seafood.

Blender: A blender is needed for making smoothies, processing ingredients for sauces and dips, and puréeing soups. Look for one that has at least 450 watts of power, which is strong enough to handle a variety of ingredients.

Assorted mixing bowls: Look for nesting bowls with lids, which can double as storage for leftovers.

Other tools: A variety of other tools will be needed for safe, efficient, and healthy cooking, including a steamer basket, a meat thermometer (an instant-read thermometer is convenient), a sieve or colander, measuring cups and spoons, a kitchen timer, pot holders, oven mitts, a vegetable peeler, spoons (slotted and wooden), a ladle, a can opener, and a whisk.

Think about adding, not subtracting, and focus on one meal or snack at a time. Pick one meal or snack you want to start with and go from there. Maybe snack time includes processed foods. Next time you shop, don't buy your usual processed snacks. Instead pick up some fresh fruit and unsalted nuts.

Nice-to-Have Equipment

If you have the resources, the following pieces of equipment take some of the work out of cooking and preparation.

Programmable pressure cooker: This is a multi-cooker that does the job of a slow cooker, electric pressure cooker, rice cooker, steamer, sauté/browning pan, and warming pot.

Food processor: Anything that can be mixed or chopped can be done in a food processor. Food processors have different sizes and types of blades, making them suitable for everything from chopping ingredients for salsa to slicing potatoes.

Toaster oven: A toaster oven is more energy efficient than a regular oven and has the ability to brown foods quickly in a way that a microwave cannot.

Step 4: Learn to Meal Plan

One of the most important keys to successfully following the DASH diet is meal planning. If that sounds overwhelming to you, rest assured, once you learn the steps, it is one of the easiest things you can do to make your life healthier and better in general, but it tends to be one of the things we neglect when life gets busy.

Meal planning is a great way to ensure you are getting a balanced diet and meeting your recommended number of servings from each food group. And as every frugal cook knows, menu planning can also save you time and money. With meal and menu planning, you know what your meals will be in advance and what you need to buy. This makes grocery shopping more efficient and cuts down on unplanned trips to the store. Meal planning also prevents the "What's for dinner?" dilemma and eliminates the need to pick up fast food on the way home from work.

The Half Plate Rule: Filling half of your plate at lunch and dinner with low-calorie vegetables not only fills you up so you don't feel deprived, but it can help you to meet the DASH recommended 4 to 5 servings of fruits and vegetables per day.

Menu planning doesn't have to be complicated, and there are a number of ways to approach it. Chapter 3 offers an easy 21-day meal plan with shopping lists to help you get started right away. You can use the menu as-is or customize it based on your preferences by interchanging recipes within the meal categories. Once you have planned your meals for several weeks, you will discover the method that works best for you and your family.

A pen, paper, and a few minutes are all you really need to get started. Once you are ready to meal plan, use this step-by-step guide to get you on your way.

1. **Plan ahead, but not too far ahead.** Typical meal-planning advice is to plan for one week of meals, and shop accordingly. Look at your schedule for the week and write down any activities that will affect your mealtimes. Next write down the total number of meals you will need to prepare for the week, including breakfast, lunch, dinner, and snacks.

2. **Shop your refrigerator and cupboards first.** Make a list of the foods you have in the refrigerator, freezer, or cupboard that need to be used up. Do you have Brussels sprouts that need to be used? Frozen fish hiding in your freezer?

3. **Mix things up.** Keep your menu interesting by planning some meatless meals or substituting a breakfast for a dinner. Alternate new recipes and old favorites. Think seasonally: What fresh produce is available this time of year?

4. **Picture your plate.** As you plan each meal, keep in mind that vegetables and fruits should cover half of your plate, lean protein should cover a quarter, and the rest of your plate should be whole grains.

5. **Plan for leftovers.** Check the serving sizes when you pick your recipes: Are you likely to have leftovers from any of your meals? If so, plan to eat leftovers one evening each week, or store them in ready-to-go lunch-size portions for the following day.

6. **Choose your recipes.** Now that you have gathered your information, reviewed your schedule, and checked your pantry, it's time to pick recipes. Select recipes with similar ingredients to minimize how much you need to buy, and consider family members' preferences.

7. **Use your meal plan to make your shopping list.** Be certain to include the exact quantities of the ingredients you need for each recipe to avoid overbuying or not buying enough. Set aside time to shop, and remember to take your list to the grocery store.

Congratulations! You are on your way to becoming a meal-planning pro. Keep in mind that your menu isn't set in stone, so be flexible and feel free to swap things around. Lastly, don't throw away your meal plan at the end of the week. Instead, hold on to it and reuse it later.

Step 5: Get Moving

Making exercise a habit can help lower your blood pressure, give you more energy, lower your stress, improve your mood, help you manage your weight, and improve your sleep. If you are not currently active, check in with your doctor first. This is especially important if you are taking medication to treat your high blood pressure; have heart disease, diabetes, or other coexisting conditions like kidney disease; and are male over the age of 40 or female over the age of 50. Only your healthcare provider can determine if you are healthy enough for exercise.

Once you receive medical clearance you can do any type of activity you like, and you don't need to go to a gym if that's not your preference. Current recommendations are to accumulate a total of 150 minutes of moderate aerobic activity or 75 minutes of vigorous aerobic activity a week, or a combination of the two. An easy way to achieve this is to aim for at least 30 minutes of activity most days of the week. If you can't set aside that much time at once, remember that short bursts of activity count, too, so you can break it up into three 10-minute sessions and get the same benefits.

5 WAYS TO DE-STRESS

Constant stress, whether from work, daily traffic, or an overloaded schedule, can have real physical effects on the body. Stress has been linked to a range of health issues including sleep disturbances, increased hunger, high blood pressure, and even heart disease. Break the connection and learn to manage your stress using these five simple tips.

1. **Breathe:** Slow, deep breathing for only a few minutes can dramatically decrease tension.

2. **Count:** Counting numbers gives the mind something neutral to focus on. This diversion can get you on a more serene track.

3. **Laugh:** Let loose with a resounding belly laugh! It will reduce levels of epinephrine, cortisol, and other stress hormones. And remember, it is the physical act of laughing that counts; nothing has to be funny to enjoy this stress-busting benefit.

4. **Pet an animal:** Merely stroking a dog or cat can trigger release of oxytocin, a hormone that helps reduce cortisol levels.

5. **Stroll in nature:** While any walk will help to clear your head and boost endorphins, walking in a park or other green space can actually put your body in a state of meditation, which allows for reflection.

Cardiovascular/Aerobic Exercise

Any physical activity that increases your heart rate and breathing rate is considered aerobic activity. Aerobic activity includes walking, swimming, bicycling (stationary or outdoor), household chores, dancing, climbing stairs, and yard work. To start being more active each day, try these simple steps:

- Take the stairs instead of the elevator.
- Take the dog on longer walks.
- Take a walk on your lunch hour.
- Get off the bus one stop earlier.
- Walk around the house (aka "housewalking").
- Carry the groceries in from the car one bag at a time.

Strength Training

Strength training builds strong muscles that help you burn more calories throughout the day. It is also important for keeping your muscles and joints healthy. Muscle-building exercises can be done with only your body weight, resistance bands, dumbbells, kettle bells, and medicine balls. A note of caution, however: Training with weights can cause a temporary increase in blood pressure during exercise, and this effect can be dramatic depending on how much you lift. Work with your doctor to assess the risks and benefits of training with weights.

Stretching, Warm-Up, Cool-Down

Stretching makes you more flexible, helps you move better, and prevents injury. Current recommendations are to do flexibility-type exercises at least two days a week to improve range of motion. Aim to stretch each major body part and hold each stretch, to the point of tightness, for 10 to 30 seconds before releasing. You can incorporate stretching as part of your warm-up and cool-down before and after you exercise. Doing a warm-up and cool-down is especially important for someone with high blood pressure.

Sample Exercise Sequences

Use the following examples as a guide for incorporating regular exercise, always starting with a warm-up and finishing with a cool-down.

- **Beginner's walking workout:** On a treadmill or outdoors, alternate very brisk walking for 1 minute, followed by moderate walking for 1 minute, repeating the circuit for a total of 10 to 30 minutes. As you build up your strength, increase the length of each interval to 2 minutes.

- **Intermediate/advanced level 20-minute interval treadmill workout:** Walk/slow jog for 1 minute at 3.5 mph at a 4 percent incline, followed by a speed walk/run for 1 minute at 4.5 mph at a 6 percent incline. Repeat the circuit for 20 minutes.

- **Bodyweight workout (any level):** Complete this circuit as many times as you can in 15 minutes—10 squats, 10 lunges on each leg, 10 pushups, and 10 crunches.

Keep This in Mind

Remember to keep perspective throughout your transition to the DASH eating plan, and take things one step at a time. Consider allowing yourself additional time for rest and relaxation to keep stress levels in check. You don't have a deadline to meet, so take the pressure off and start with a few DASH meals or snacks per week, pick out some recipes to try, and make use of the 21-day plan provided in the next chapter. Think about your current meals and snacks and how you can *add* to them to make them more "DASH-friendly." And when a meal or snack works, write it down so you can recycle it and repeat your successes. Lastly, continue to celebrate each step you take in your journey to a healthier you.

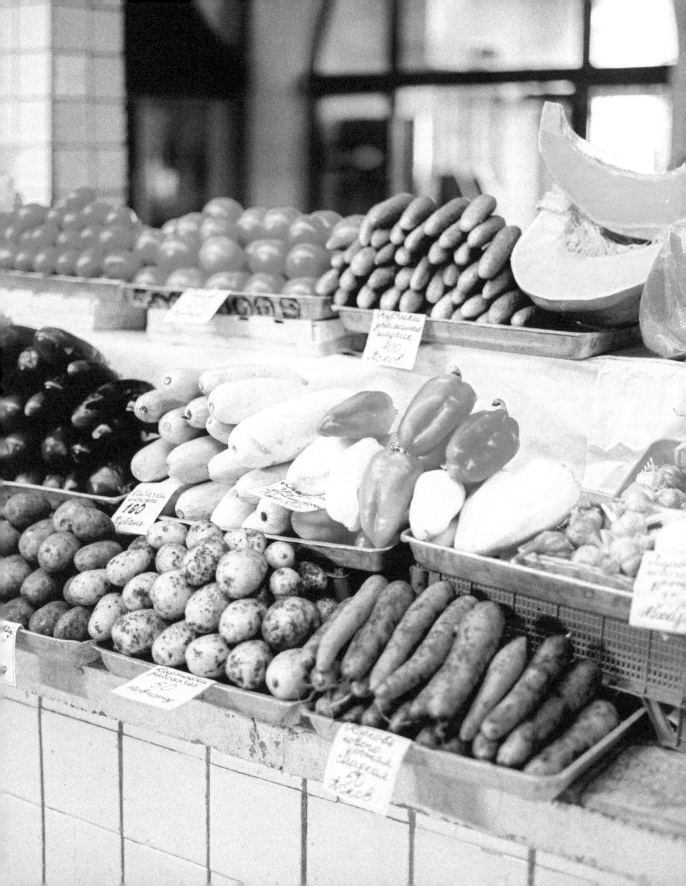

CHAPTER

3

The Plan

As you've learned, the DASH diet is an excellent eating plan high in important nutrients, including calcium, potassium, magnesium, lean protein, and fiber, and it's low in sodium. To help you get started with the DASH diet, this chapter contains a 21-day sample DASH meal plan complete with weekly shopping lists and a basic pantry list.

The shopping list for each week is written for two people, so adjust for more or less as needed. If a suggested meal or snack doesn't appeal to you, simply make a DASH-friendly substitute using the recipes in this book. If you adjust the menu, be certain to also adjust the shopping list.

Keep in mind that DASH is an eating plan that focuses on your overall dietary pattern over the course of a few days or a week. So if you don't follow the plan exactly and have more servings of a food on one day and less on another, you can still meet the requirements set out by DASH. The one exception is sodium, which you should aim to keep between 1,500 mg and 2,300 mg on a daily basis. The following menus are intended as a guide only, and you may need a higher or a lower number of servings based on your individual calorie needs.

Week One Meal Plan

Suggested Menu

*Meals in blue are recipes from this book. Use the other meal suggestions as a guide, or swap out with recipes in this book. To boost your dairy intake, depending on your daily calorie needs, have a glass of nonfat or low-fat milk with one or more of your meals.

Sunday

BREAKFAST Greek Yogurt Oat Pancakes (page 51)

SNACK 1 medium-size piece of fruit

LUNCH 3 ounces grilled chicken, 1 cup steamed vegetables, ½ cup brown rice

SNACK 1 stick light string cheese, 1 medium-size piece of fruit

DINNER Salmon and Asparagus in Foil (page 96)

Monday

BREAKFAST 2 slices whole-grain toast with 1 ounce nonfat/low-fat cheese, 2 boiled eggs, 1 banana

SNACK 1 medium-size piece of fruit

LUNCH Leftover Salmon and Asparagus in Foil

SNACK 1 cup nonfat or low-fat plain Greek or regular yogurt, 1 medium-size piece of fruit

DINNER Spicy Bean Chili (page 62)

Tuesday

BREAKFAST Creamy Apple-Avocado Smoothie (page 48)

SNACK 1 medium-size piece of fruit

LUNCH Leftover Spicy Bean Chili

SNACK 1 cup nonfat or low-fat milk, 1 ounce unsalted nuts

DINNER Apricot Chicken (page 92)

Wednesday

BREAKFAST ¾ cup bran flakes cereal with 2 tablespoons nuts, 8 ounces nonfat or low-fat milk, 1 banana

SNACK 1 medium-size piece of fruit

LUNCH Leftover Apricot Chicken

SNACK ½ cup nonfat or low-fat cottage cheese, 1 medium-size piece of fruit

DINNER Halibut with Greens and Ginger (page 98)

Thursday

BREAKFAST Stuffed Breakfast Peppers (page 54)

SNACK 1 medium-size piece of fruit

LUNCH Leftover Halibut with Greens and Ginger

SNACK 1 cup nonfat or low-fat plain Greek or regular yogurt, 1 medium-size piece of fruit

DINNER Ground Turkey–Brussels Sprouts Skillet (page 89)

Friday

BREAKFAST 1 cup oatmeal with 1 cup nonfat or low-fat milk, 1 cup raspberries

SNACK 1 medium-size piece of fruit

LUNCH Leftover Ground Turkey–Brussels Sprouts Skillet

SNACK 1 ounce unsalted nuts, 1 medium-size piece of fruit

DINNER Steak with Chickpeas and Spinach (page 126)

Saturday

BREAKFAST Leftover Stuffed Breakfast Peppers

SNACK 1 medium-size piece of fruit

LUNCH Leftover Steak with Chickpeas and Spinach

SNACK 1 cup nonfat or low-fat milk, 1 medium-size piece of fruit

DINNER 4 ounces grilled fish, 1 cup steamed vegetables, baked sweet potato, ½ cup nonfat or low-fat cottage cheese

Pantry List

Check your pantry for olive oil, nonstick cooking spray, pepper, garlic, onions, rolled oats, unsalted peanut butter, unsalted almonds, nonfat or low-fat milk, fresh fruit, and salad greens.

Week One Shopping List

Canned and Bottled Items

- Chicken stock, no salt (4 ounces)
- Chickpeas (1 [15-ounce] can)
- Kidney beans (2 [15-ounce] cans)
- Lime juice (1 tablespoon)
- Tomatoes, no-salt (1 [8-ounce] can)
- Vegetable broth, low-sodium (8 ounces)

Dairy and Eggs

- Cheese, low-fat (2 ounces)
- Cheese, shredded, low-fat (¼ cup)
- Cottage cheese, low-fat (16 ounces)
- Egg whites, liquid (1 small container)
- Eggs (1 dozen)
- Greek yogurt, vanilla, nonfat (8 ounces)
- Greek yogurt, plain, nonfat or low-fat (40 ounces)
- Milk, nonfat or low-fat (½ gallon)
- String cheese, low-fat (2 sticks)

Frozen

- Spinach (1 [16-ounce] bag)
- Vegetables, mixed (1 [16-ounce] bag)

Meat

- Chicken breasts, boneless (6)
- Fish fillets of choice (2 [4-ounce] fillets)
- Halibut fillets (4 [4-ounce] fillets)
- Salmon fillets (4 [5-ounce] fillets)
- Steak, flank (12 ounces)
- Turkey, ground, 93% lean white meat (1 pound)

Pantry Items

- Baking powder
- Balsamic vinegar (1 tablespoon)
- Black pepper
- Bread, whole-grain (4 slices)
- Brown rice (1 cup)
- Cereal, breakfast, whole-grain bran (10-ounce box)
- Chili powder
- Cinnamon, ground
- Dill, dried
- Honey (¼ cup)
- Nuts, unsalted (5 ounces)
- Oats, rolled (2 cups)
- Thyme, dried

Produce

- Apple (1)
- Apricots (8)
- Asparagus (1 pound)
- Avocado (1)
- Baby spinach (13 cups)
- Bananas (4)
- Bell peppers (5)
- Brussels sprouts (½ pound)
- Fruit (14 medium-size pieces; can also use canned in light syrup or unsweetened dried fruit)
- Garlic cloves (8)
- Gingerroot (1 piece)
- Lemons (2)
- Mint, fresh (¼ cup)
- Onions, red, medium (2)
- Orange (1)
- Raspberries (2 cups)
- Scallions (2)
- Sweet potatoes (2)

Other

- White wine, dry (½ cup)

Week Two Meal Plan

Suggested Menu

*Meals in blue are recipes from this book. Use the other meal suggestions as a guide, or swap out with recipes in this book. To boost your dairy intake, depending on your daily calorie needs, have a glass of nonfat or low-fat milk with one or more of your meals.

Sunday

BREAKFAST Steel-Cut Oatmeal with Plums and Pear (page 59)

SNACK 1 medium-size piece of fruit

LUNCH 4 ounces grilled fish, 2 cups mixed greens, ½ cup brown rice

SNACK ½ cup nonfat or low-fat cottage cheese, ½ cup fruit

DINNER Pasta Primavera (page 67)

Monday

BREAKFAST 2 hardboiled eggs, 1 cup oats, 1 banana

SNACK 1 medium-size piece of fruit

LUNCH Leftover Pasta Primavera

SNACK 1 cup nonfat or low-fat plain Greek or regular yogurt, 1 medium-size piece of fruit

DINNER Red Lentil Stew (page 66)

Tuesday

BREAKFAST Leftover Steel-Cut Oatmeal with Plums and Pear

SNACK 1 medium-size piece of fruit

LUNCH Leftover Red Lentil Stew

SNACK 1 ounce unsalted nuts, 1 hardboiled egg

DINNER Tandoori Chicken with Rice (page 91)

Wednesday

BREAKFAST Blueberry-Vanilla Yogurt Smoothie (page 50)

SNACK 1 medium-size piece of fruit

LUNCH Leftover Tandoori Chicken with Rice

SNACK 1 stick light string cheese, 1 medium-size piece of fruit

DINNER Baked Flounder Packets with Summer Squash (page 100)

Thursday

BREAKFAST 2 slices whole-grain toast with 2 tablespoons nut butter, 1 apple, 1 glass nonfat or low-fat milk

SNACK 1 medium-size piece of fruit

LUNCH Leftover Baked Flounder Packets with Summer Squash

SNACK 1 cup nonfat or low-fat plain Greek or regular yogurt, 1 medium-size piece of fruit

DINNER Chickpea Burgers (page 70) with 2 cups mixed greens

Friday

BREAKFAST Apple-Apricot Brown Rice Breakfast Porridge (page 57)

SNACK 1 medium-size piece of fruit

LUNCH Leftover Chickpea Burgers with 2 cups mixed greens

SNACK ½ cup nonfat or low-fat cottage cheese, ½ cup fruit

DINNER Pistachio-Crusted Chicken (page 94)

Saturday

BREAKFAST Leftover Apple-Apricot Brown Rice Breakfast Porridge

SNACK 1 medium-size piece of fruit

LUNCH Leftover Pistachio-Crusted Chicken

SNACK 1 stick light string cheese, 1 ounce unsalted nuts

DINNER 3 ounces pork fillet, 1 cup mixed vegetables, 1 cup brown rice

Pantry List

Compare this week's shopping list with the previous list and cross off anything you purchased the week before. Specifically, check your pantry for olive oil, nonstick cooking spray, pepper, garlic, onions, rolled oats, unsalted peanut butter, unsalted almonds, nonfat or low-fat milk, fresh fruit, and salad greens.

Week Two Shopping List

Canned and Bottled Items

- Chickpeas (1 [15-ounce] can)
- Evaporated milk, fat-free
  (1 [8-ounce] can)
- Tomatoes, diced, no salt
  (1 [14-ounce] can)
- Vegetable broth, low-sodium (5 cups)
- Lemon juice

Dairy and Eggs

- Cottage cheese, low-fat (16 ounces)
- Eggs (½ dozen)
- Greek yogurt, vanilla,
  nonfat (8 ounces)
- Greek yogurt, plain,
  nonfat (24 ounces)
- Milk, nonfat (1 gallon)
- Parmesan cheese, fresh (4 ounces)
- String cheese, low-fat (4 sticks)

Frozen

- Blueberries (12 ounces)
- Vegetables, mixed (1 [16-ounce] bag)

Meat

- Chicken breasts, boneless,
  skinless (2 pounds, about 4)
- Fish fillets of choice
  (2 [4-ounce] fillets)
- Flounder fillets (4 [6-ounce] fillets)
- Pork fillet, lean (6 ounces)

Pantry Items

- Almonds (¼ cup)
- Angel-hair pasta, whole-wheat (8 ounces)
- Apricots, dried (4)
- Basil, dried
- Bread, whole-grain (4 slices)
- Brown rice (2½ cups)
- Brown rice, instant (1 cup)
- Cinnamon, ground
- Cumin
- Curry powder
- Garlic powder
- Ginger, ground
- Lentils, dried (1 cup)
- Nuts of choice, unsalted (4 ounces)
- Oats, rolled (3 cups)
- Oats, steel-cut (1 cup)
- Onion powder
- Paprika
- Pistachio nuts (½ cup)
- Plums, dried (prunes) (1 cup)
- Sage, dried
- Vanilla extract
- Walnuts (½ cup)

Produce

- Apples (2)
- Bananas (3)
- Baby salad greens, mixed (12 cups)
- Broccoli florets (2 cups)
- Carrots (3)
- Fruit (14 medium pieces; can also use canned in light syrup or unsweetened dried fruit)
- Garlic gloves (7)
- Lemon (1)
- Mushrooms (1 cup)
- Onions (3)
- Parsley, fresh (⅓ cup)
- Pear (1)
- Summer squash (3)
- Zucchini (2)

Week Three Meal Plan

Suggested Menu

*Meals in blue are recipes from this book. Use the other meal suggestions as a guide, or swap out with recipes in this book. To boost your dairy intake, depending on your daily calorie needs, have a glass of nonfat or low-fat milk with one or more of your meals.

Sunday

BREAKFAST Scrambled Egg and Veggie Breakfast Quesadillas (page 52)

SNACK 1 medium-size piece of fruit

LUNCH 3 ounces grilled chicken breast, 2 cups baby greens, 2 tablespoons walnuts

SNACK 1 cup nonfat or low-fat plain Greek or regular yogurt, 1 medium-size piece of fruit

DINNER Pecan-Crusted Catfish (page 102)

Monday

BREAKFAST 1 cup oatmeal, ¾ cup nonfat or low-fat Greek or regular yogurt, 1 banana

SNACK 1 medium-size piece of fruit

LUNCH Leftover Pecan-Crusted Catfish

SNACK 1 stick light string cheese, 1 ounce unsalted nuts

DINNER White Bean and Roasted Red Pepper Soup (page 64)

Tuesday

BREAKFAST Creamy Apple-Avocado Smoothie (page 48)

SNACK 1 medium-size piece of fruit

LUNCH Leftover White Bean and Roasted Red Pepper Soup

SNACK string cheese, 1 ounce unsalted nuts, 1 cup berries

DINNER Spiced Lentils and Poached Eggs (page 76)

Wednesday

BREAKFAST 2 slices whole-grain toast, 2 tablespoons nut butter, 1 cup nonfat or low-fat milk, 1 banana

SNACK 1 medium-size piece of fruit

LUNCH Leftover Spiced Lentils and Poached Eggs

SNACK 1 cup nonfat or low-fat plain Greek or regular yogurt, 1 ounce unsalted nuts

DINNER Chicken Legs with Rice and Peas (page 103)

Thursday

BREAKFAST Stuffed Breakfast Peppers (page 54)

SNACK 1 medium-size piece of fruit

LUNCH Leftover Chicken Legs with Rice and Peas

SNACK 1 stick light string cheese, 1 medium-size piece of fruit

DINNER Mexican Beans and Rice (page 73)

Friday

BREAKFAST Carrot Cake Overnight Oats (page 58)

SNACK 1 medium-size piece of fruit

LUNCH Leftover Mexican Beans and Rice

SNACK ½ piece of fruit, low-fat plain Greek yogurt or regular yogurt, 1 medium-size piece of fruit

DINNER Spinach-Stuffed Turkey Burgers (page 88)

Saturday

BREAKFAST Leftover Stuffed Breakfast Peppers

SNACK 1 medium-size piece of fruit

LUNCH Leftover Spinach-Stuffed Turkey Burgers

SNACK 1 cup nonfat or low-fat plain Greek or regular yogurt, 1 medium-size piece of fruit

DINNER 4 ounces grilled fish fillet, 1 sweet potato, 1 cup mixed vegetables

Pantry List

Compare this week's shopping list with the previous list and cross off anything you purchased the week before. Specifically, check your pantry for olive oil, nonstick cooking spray, pepper, garlic, onions, rolled oats, unsalted peanut butter, unsalted almonds, nonfat or low fat milk, fresh fruit, and salad greens.

Week Three Shopping List

Canned and Bottled Items

- Black beans (2 [15-ounce] cans)
- Cannellini beans (1 [15-ounce] can)
- Lemon juice
- Tomatoes, diced, no-salt (1 [14.5-ounce] can)
- Vegetable broth, low-sodium (2 cups)

Dairy and Eggs

- Cheese, shredded, low-fat (¼ cup)
- Cottage cheese, low-fat (16 ounces)
- Eggs (1 dozen)
- Greek yogurt, plain, nonfat (32 ounces, plus 24 ounces)
- Greek yogurt, vanilla, nonfat (8 ounces)
- Milk, nonfat (1 quart)
- String cheese, low-fat (4 sticks)

Frozen

- Peas (1 [16-ounce] bag)
- Spinach (1 [16-ounce] bag)
- Vegetables, mixed (1 [16-ounce] bag)

Meat

- Catfish fillets (4 [4-ounce] fillets)
- Chicken breast (6 ounces)
- Chicken drumsticks (4)
- Fish fillets of choice (2 [4-ounce] fillets)
- Turkey, ground, 93% lean white meat (12 ounces)

Pantry Items

- Bread, whole-grain (4 slices)
- Brown rice (1½ cups)
- Chili powder
- Corn tortillas (4)
- Cumin
- Curry powder
- Garlic powder
- Lentils, dried (1 cup)
- Nuts, unsalted (2 ounces)
- Oats, rolled (2½ cups)
- Oregano, dried
- Pecans (¾ cup)
- Raisins (¼ cup)
- Rosemary, dried
- Walnuts (1 ounce)
- White vinegar

Produce

- Apple (1)
- Avocados (2)
- Baby greens, mixed (4 cups)
- Baby spinach (5 cups)
- Bananas (4)
- Carrot, shredded (½ cup)
- Cilantro, fresh (1 bunch)
- Fruit (14 medium pieces; can also use canned in light syrup or unsweetened dried fruit)
- Garlic cloves (14)
- Jalapeño pepper (1)
- Lemons (2)
- Onions (2)
- Oregano, fresh (1 bunch)
- Red peppers (3)
- Sweet potatoes (2)
- Tomatoes (2)

About the Recipes

All of the recipes in this part yield from one to four servings. They call for readily available ingredients that are both nutritious and economical. The ingredients have been selected for their blood pressure–lowering nutrients, including calcium, potassium, magnesium, B vitamins, and plant nutrients (aka phytonutrients). The recipes are also high in fiber, vitamins, and minerals, and low in sodium and saturated fat. Nutrition information is included for each recipe so you can keep track. When an ingredient choice is offered, the nutrition information reflects the first one. When you include an optional ingredient in your recipe, be sure to add it to your total counts.

The labels included with each recipe help you quickly identify if a particular recipe is right for you. Here is what each label indicates.

Vegan: Recipes do not contain any animal products.

Veggie: Recipes contain dairy and/or eggs but no other animal products.

30-Min: The dish can be prepared in 30 minutes or less.

1-Pot: The recipe requires only one pot, baking sheet, or other type of kitchen equipment, such as a blender or a jar.

$-Saver: The main ingredients in the recipe cost around $5, and the recipe allows for the use of frozen, canned, and dried ingredients.

PART 2

Recipes for DASH Living

Creamy Apple-
Avocado Smoothie,
page 48

Breakfasts & Smoothies

Creamy Apple-Avocado Smoothie

SERVES 2 • PREP TIME: 5 MINUTES

This thick and creamy green smoothie offers a host of blood pressure–lowering benefits. Avocados are rich in monounsaturated fatty acids, which are plant-based fats that enhance heart health. Apples are high in vitamin C and cholesterol-lowering fiber and are a rich source of potassium, giving this treat an extra hypertension-lowering punch. With a sweet and earthy taste, it is as filling as it is nutritious.

½ medium avocado, peeled and pitted

1 medium apple, chopped

1 cup baby spinach leaves

1 cup nonfat vanilla Greek yogurt

½ to 1 cup water

1 cup ice

Freshly squeezed lemon juice (optional)

1. In a blender, combine all of the ingredients, and blend until smooth and creamy.

2. Top with a squeeze of fresh lemon juice if desired, and serve immediately.

BUDGET-SAVER TIP Frozen spinach can be more economical than fresh, and frozen will make your smoothie thicker. If using frozen, reduce the quantity to ½ cup.

Nutrition (per serving) Calories: 200; Total Fat: 7g; Saturated Fat: 1g; Cholesterol: 5mg; Sodium: 56mg; Potassium: 378mg; Magnesium: 16mg; Total Carbohydrates: 27g; Fiber: 5g; Sugars: 20g; Protein: 10g

Strawberry, Orange, and Beet Smoothie

SERVES 2 • PREP TIME: 5 MINUTES

This smoothie combines the blood pressure–lowering power of nonfat milk, beets, strawberries, and oranges in a creamy and sweet fiber-rich meal in a glass. Milk and yogurt contain calcium and vitamin D, two nutrients that work together to reduce blood pressure, while beets are a rich source of nitrates, which open up your blood vessels to help lower pressure. Sweet and filling, this smoothie is also a great source of vitamins A and C, and the minerals potassium and magnesium.

1 cup nonfat milk

1 cup frozen strawberries

1 medium beet, cooked, peeled, and cubed

1 orange, peeled and quartered

1 frozen banana, peeled and chopped

1 cup nonfat vanilla Greek yogurt

1 cup ice

1. In a blender, combine all of the ingredients, and blend until smooth and creamy.

2. Serve immediately.

INGREDIENT TIP When you have overripe bananas, slice them and freeze them for use in smoothies. Frozen bananas add sweetness, eliminating the need for added sugar. They also make smoothies thick and creamy and add valuable amounts of the blood pressure–lowering mineral potassium.

Nutrition (per serving) Calories: 266; Total Fat: 0g; Saturated Fat: 0g; Cholesterol: 7mg; Sodium: 104mg; Potassium: 731mg; Magnesium: 40mg; Total Carbohydrates: 51g; Fiber: 6g; Sugars: 34g; Protein: 15g

Blueberry-Vanilla Yogurt Smoothie

SERVES 2 • PREP TIME: 5 MINUTES

Blueberries may very well be one of the keys to good health. High in inflammation-reducing antioxidants and blood pressure–lowering nitrates, blueberries are also a good source of fiber and vitamin C. Rich in potassium, calcium, vitamin D, and probiotics, this smoothie is good at breakfast and as an afternoon snack.

1½ cups
frozen blueberries

1 cup nonfat vanilla
Greek yogurt

1 frozen banana,
peeled and sliced

½ cup nonfat or
low-fat milk

1 cup ice

1. In a blender, combine all of the ingredients, and blend until smooth and creamy.

2. Serve immediately.

INGREDIENT TIP To keep costs in check, take advantage of blueberry season and freeze several bags of berries for use throughout the year. Fresh blueberries can be washed and frozen whole without damaging their antioxidant content; just be certain to drain the berries thoroughly before freezing.

Nutrition (per serving) Calories: 228; Total Fat: 1g; Saturated Fat: 0g; Cholesterol: 6mg; Sodium: 63mg; Potassium: 470mg; Magnesium: 32mg; Total Carbohydrates: 45g; Fiber: 5g; Sugars: 34g; Protein: 12g

Greek Yogurt Oat Pancakes

SERVES 2 • PREP TIME: 5 MINUTES • COOK TIME: 10 MINUTES

You might think pancakes are off-limits when you are following a heart-healthy diet. However, a few nutrient-rich replacements is all it takes to transform a high-calorie starchy breakfast into a protein-packed meal high in cholesterol-lowering fiber and blood pressure–lowering vitamins and minerals. Easy to make, these are perfect for a weekday morning.

6 egg whites
(or ¾ cup liquid
egg whites)

1 cup rolled oats

1 cup plain nonfat
Greek yogurt

1 medium banana,
peeled and sliced

1 teaspoon ground
cinnamon

1 teaspoon
baking powder

1. In a blender, combine all of the ingredients and blend until smooth. For best results, allow the batter to sit and thicken while the griddle is heating, about 5 minutes.

2. Heat a griddle or large nonstick skillet over medium heat. Spray the skillet with nonstick cooking spray.

3. Pour about one-third cup of the batter onto the griddle. Allow to cook, and flip when bubbles on top burst, about 5 minutes. Cook for another couple of minutes until golden brown. Repeat with the remaining batter.

4. Divide between two serving plates and enjoy.

SUBSTITUTION TIP Although Greek yogurt is higher in protein and lower in sodium and sugar than regular yogurt, regular yogurt actually contains slightly more calcium and potassium. It is also generally less expensive. Both types of yogurt are a healthy choice.

Nutrition (per serving) Calories: 318; Total Fat: 4g; Saturated Fat: 0g; Cholesterol: 5mg; Sodium: 467mg; Potassium: 634mg; Magnesium: 20mg; Total Carbohydrates: 47g; Fiber: 6g; Sugars: 13g; Protein: 28g

Scrambled Egg and Veggie Breakfast Quesadillas

SERVES 2 • PREP TIME: 15 MINUTES • COOK TIME: 15 MINUTES

A breakfast quesadilla is a great choice when you want to get a jump-start on your recommended servings of several food groups, including fruits, veggies, beans, grains, and lean protein. This dish is made with fluffy scrambled eggs mixed with black beans and tomatoes and topped with fresh cilantro and avocado. Corn tortillas are lower in calories than their wheat counterparts; they also have more fiber, magnesium, and potassium, and less sodium.

2 eggs

2 egg whites

2 to 4 tablespoons nonfat or low-fat milk

¼ teaspoon freshly ground black pepper

1 large tomato, chopped

2 tablespoons chopped cilantro

½ cup canned black beans, rinsed and drained

1½ tablespoons olive oil, divided

4 corn tortillas

½ avocado, peeled, pitted, and thinly sliced

1. In a bowl, combine the eggs, egg whites, milk, and black pepper. Using an electric mixer, beat until smooth. To the same bowl, add the tomato, cilantro, and black beans, and fold into the eggs with a spoon.

2. Heat half of the olive oil in a medium pan over medium heat. Add the scrambled-egg mixture and cook for a few minutes, stirring, until cooked through. Remove from the pan.

3. Divide the scrambled-egg mixture between the tortillas, layering only on one half of the tortilla.

4. Top with avocado slices and fold the tortillas in half.

5. Heat the remaining oil over medium heat, and add one of the folded tortillas to the pan. Cook for 1 to 2 minutes on each side, or until browned. Repeat with remaining tortillas.

6. Serve immediately.

INGREDIENT TIP Cilantro is a good source of the minerals potassium, calcium, and magnesium, all of which are nutrients important for blood-pressure regulation. Cilantro is very low in calories, inexpensive, and available year-round. Consider making it a regular addition to your diet.

Nutrition (per serving) Calories: 445; Total Fat: 24g; Saturated Fat: 4g; Cholesterol: 186mg; Sodium: 228mg; Potassium: 614mg; Magnesium: 64mg; Total Carbohydrates: 42g; Fiber: 11g; Sugars: 2g; Protein: 19g

Stuffed Breakfast Peppers

SERVES 4 • PREP TIME: 5 MINUTES • COOK TIME: 35 TO 45 MINUTES

A rival to their stuffed-avocado counterpart, stuffed peppers make a filling breakfast that is rich in protein, vitamins, and minerals. Bell peppers are very high in the antioxidant vitamin C—one pepper contains about 169 percent of the RDA. Also a good source of fiber and the mineral potassium, peppers are low in calories, which makes them an excellent addition to a DASH-style eating plan.

4 bell peppers
(any color)

1 (16-ounce) bag
frozen spinach

4 eggs

¼ cup shredded
low-fat cheese
(optional)

Freshly ground
black pepper

1. Preheat the oven to 400°F. Line a baking dish with aluminum foil.

2. Slice the tops off each pepper and remove the seeds. Discard the tops and seeds.

3. Place the peppers in the baking dish, and bake for about 15 minutes.

4. While the peppers bake, defrost the spinach and drain off the excess moisture.

5. Remove the peppers from the oven and stuff the bottoms evenly with the defrosted spinach.

6. Crack an egg over the spinach inside each pepper. Top each egg with a tablespoon of the cheese (if using), and season with black pepper, to taste.

7. Bake for about 15 to 20 minutes, or until the egg whites are set and opaque.

INGREDIENT TIP When selecting peppers, look for ones that are wrinkle-free, shiny, and unblemished. Peppers should be firm when you buy them. Red peppers are simply mature green peppers; yellow and orange peppers are different, sweeter varieties.

Nutrition (per serving) Calories: 136; Total Fat: 5g; Saturated Fat: 2g; Cholesterol: 186mg; Sodium: 131mg; Potassium: 576mg; Magnesium: 80mg; Total Carbohydrates: 15g; Fiber: 5g; Sugars: 3g; Protein: 11g

Sweet Potato Toast Three Ways

SERVES 2 • PREP TIME: 10 MINUTES • COOK TIME: 5 MINUTES

If you haven't tried sweet-potato toast yet, now is the time to put down your wheat toast and trade it for this potassium- and fiber-rich breakfast alternative. Not only do sweet potatoes taste like dessert, but they also have so many health benefits that it's hard to list them all. An outstanding source of the antioxidant beta-carotene, one cup of this nutritious veggie has over 200 percent of the RDA of vitamin A. The trickiest part of making sweet-potato toast is ensuring that each slice gets toasted long enough to cook through.

1 large sweet potato, unpeeled

TOPPING CHOICE #1

4 tablespoons peanut butter

1 ripe banana, sliced

Dash ground cinnamon

TOPPING CHOICE #2

½ avocado, peeled, pitted, and mashed

2 eggs (1 per slice)

TOPPING CHOICE #3

4 tablespoons nonfat or low-fat ricotta cheese

1 tomato, sliced

Dash black pepper

1. Slice the sweet potato lengthwise into ¼-inch thick slices.

2. Place the sweet potato slices in a toaster on high for about 5 minutes or until cooked through. Repeat multiple times, if necessary, depending on your toaster settings.

3. Top with your desired topping choices and enjoy.

INGREDIENT TIP Sweet potato toast slices can be stored in an airtight glass container for up to one week. The possibilities for toppings are endless, so use your imagination and experiment with your favorite choices.

Nutrition (per serving) (1 [5-inch] sweet potato without toppings) Calories: 137; Total Fat: 0g; Saturated Fat: 0g; Cholesterol: 0mg; Sodium: 17mg; Potassium: 265mg; Magnesium: 16mg; Total Carbohydrates: 32g; Fiber: 4g; Sugars: 0g; Protein: 2g

Apple-Apricot Brown Rice Breakfast Porridge

SERVES 4 • PREP TIME: 2 MINUTES • COOK TIME: 8 MINUTES

This creamy and delicious breakfast porridge contains a mix of powerful blood pressure–lowering foods. Apricots are an excellent source of potassium, while apples contain cholesterol-lowering fiber. Plus, brown rice is rich in magnesium, B vitamins, fiber, and numerous phytonutrients, including lignans, which protect against heart disease. Prepared with a handful of pantry staples, this recipe is quick to prepare.

3 cups cooked brown rice

1¾ cups nonfat or low-fat milk

2 tablespoons lightly packed brown sugar

4 dried apricots, chopped

1 medium apple, cored, and diced

¾ teaspoon ground cinnamon

¾ teaspoon vanilla extract

1. Combine the rice, milk, sugar, apricots, apple, and cinnamon in a medium saucepan. Bring to a boil over medium heat, then turn the heat down slightly and cook, stirring frequently, for 2 to 3 minutes or until the porridge reaches desired thickness.

2. Turn off the heat and stir in the vanilla extract.

3. Serve warm.

INGREDIENT TIP This recipe is good to use when you have leftover brown rice. If you don't have cooked brown rice on hand, prepare a batch of instant brown rice, which has the same nutrition profile as long-grain brown rice. Instant rice has simply been cooked and dehydrated.

Nutrition (per serving) Calories: 260; Total Fat: 2g; Saturated Fat: 0g; Cholesterol: 2mg; Sodium: 50mg; Potassium: 421mg; Magnesium: 20mg; Total Carbohydrates: 57g; Fiber: 4g; Sugars: 22g; Protein: 7g

Carrot Cake Overnight Oats

SERVES 1 • PREP TIME: 5 MINUTES • CHILL TIME: 8 HOURS OR OVERNIGHT

This carrot-cake oatmeal is the perfect blend of whole grains and protein to fuel you through a busy morning. Whole-grain oats contain cholesterol-lowering fiber, and carrots are high in potassium and beta-carotene, nutrients shown to be effective in lowering blood pressure. With all the sweet flavor of real carrot cake, this easy recipe will have you looking forward to breakfast.

½ cup rolled oats

½ cup plain nonfat or low-fat Greek yogurt

½ cup nonfat or low-fat milk

¼ cup shredded carrot

2 tablespoons raisins

½ teaspoon ground cinnamon

1 to 2 tablespoons chopped walnuts (optional)

1. Combine all of the ingredients in a lidded jar, shake well, and refrigerate overnight.

2. Enjoy cold, or heat in the microwave for 1 to 2 minutes or on the stovetop for 2 to 3 minutes, or until bubbling.

INGREDIENT TIP You can swap the rolled oats for steel-cut oats in this recipe as both contain nearly identical nutritional profiles. Rolled oats will soak up the liquid for a smoother, silkier texture, while steel-cut oats will have a chewier, heartier texture.

Nutrition (per serving) Calories: 331; Total Fat: 3g; Saturated Fat: 0g; Cholesterol: 7mg; Sodium: 141mg; Potassium: 557mg; Magnesium: 20mg; Total Carbohydrates: 59g; Fiber: 8g; Sugars: 26g; Protein: 22g

Steel-Cut Oatmeal with Plums and Pear

SERVES 4 • PREP TIME: 5 MINUTES • COOK TIME: 25 MINUTES

This nourishing recipe for steel-cut oats uses budget-friendly and heart-healthy dried plums (also called prunes). Dried plums are packed with nutrition; they have high levels of blood pressure–lowering potassium and magnesium, plus plenty of fiber to promote regularity. With the addition of healthy fats from the almonds and even more fiber and nutrients from the fresh pear, this breakfast will fuel you for hours.

2 cups water

1 cup nonfat or low-fat milk

1 cup steel-cut oats

1 cup dried plums, chopped

1 medium pear, cored, and skin removed, diced

4 tablespoons almonds, roughly chopped

1. Combine the water, milk, and oats in a medium pot and bring to a boil over high heat. Reduce the heat and cover. Simmer for about 10 minutes, stirring occasionally.

2. Add the plums and pear, and cover. Simmer for another 10 minutes.

3. Turn off the heat and let stand for 5 minutes until all of the liquid is absorbed.

4. To serve, top each portion with a sprinkling of almonds.

INGREDIENT TIP Sunsweet has a product called Amaz!n Diced Prunes, which are recipe-ready prunes that are diced and ready to be tossed into cereal, oatmeal, salads, or your favorite recipe. Keep some on hand for boosting the potassium and fiber content of any recipe. They also make a great snack.

Nutrition (per serving) Calories: 307; Total Fat: 6g; Saturated Fat: 1g; Cholesterol: 1mg; Sodium: 132mg; Potassium: 640mg; Magnesium: 104mg; Total Carbohydrates: 58g; Fiber: 9g; Sugars: 24g; Protein: 9g

Enchiladas with Bean Medley, page 84

CHAPTER 5

Vegetarian
& Vegan Entrées

Spicy Bean Chili

SERVES 4 • PREP TIME: 15 MINUTES • COOK TIME: 20 MINUTES

This spicy vegan chili is loaded with vegetable goodness, including onions, kidney beans, and canned tomatoes. Nutritious, versatile, and budget-friendly, kidney beans are chock-full of soluble fiber, magnesium, and potassium—nutrients that are excellent for lowering blood pressure and improving overall heart health. With just 20 minutes of cooking time, this chili fits perfectly into the DASH diet.

2 teaspoons olive oil

1 medium red onion, thinly sliced

2 garlic cloves, minced

2 (15-ounce) cans kidney beans, drained and rinsed

1 (8-ounce) can no-salt crushed tomatoes

1 cup low-sodium vegetable broth

½ cup water

2 teaspoons chili powder

¼ teaspoon ground cinnamon

1. Heat the olive oil in a large saucepan over medium-high heat. Add the onion and sauté until the onion is lightly caramelized, about 5 minutes. Add the garlic and sauté until fragrant, about 30 seconds.

2. Stir in the remaining ingredients and bring to a boil on high for 1 minute. Cover, reduce heat to low, and simmer until flavors are well combined, about 10 minutes.

3. Enjoy immediately.

INGREDIENT TIP When tomatoes are processed to create the canned version, it makes the carotenoid lycopene in the tomatoes more available to your body. Lycopene is a powerful plant chemical associated with a lower risk of prostate, lung, and stomach cancers. Be certain to choose the no-salt-added variety.

Nutrition (per serving) Calories: 223; Total Fat: 4g; Saturated Fat: 0g; Cholesterol: 0mg; Sodium: 237mg; Potassium: 170mg; Magnesium: 57mg; Total Carbohydrates: 37g; Fiber: 13g; Sugars: 1g; Protein: 12g

Herbed Mushroom Rice

SERVES 4 • PREP TIME: 10 MINUTES • COOK TIME: 15 MINUTES

This simple and delicious recipe features several foods with natural blood pressure–lowering abilities. Just a half cup of button mushrooms contains 423 mg of potassium for a mere 8 calories. Lima beans are a good source of fiber and protein, and are high in potassium.

2 teaspoons olive oil

12 ounces sliced mushrooms

3 scallion stalks, thinly sliced and separated

¾ teaspoon freshly ground black pepper

2 cups water

1 teaspoon dried rosemary

1 cup dry instant brown rice

2 cups frozen lima beans

¼ cup shredded Romano cheese (optional)

1. Heat the olive oil in a large saucepan over medium-high heat. Add the mushrooms, the white parts of the scallions, and the black pepper and sauté until the mushrooms are just cooked through, about 5 minutes.

2. Add the water and rosemary, and bring to a boil over high heat. Stir in the rice, lima beans, and half of the green parts of the scallions, and reduce the heat to medium. Cook, stirring occasionally, for 6 to 8 minutes, or until the rice is cooked and the lima beans are tender.

3. Sprinkle each serving with cheese (if using) and the remaining green parts of the scallions. Serve immediately.

SUBSTITUTION TIP You can use any type of mushrooms you like in this recipe, but if your budget allows, consider opting for shiitakes. Shiitake mushrooms have some notable health benefits, including a type of phytonutrient shown to keep cells from sticking to blood vessel walls, which maintains healthy blood pressure and improves circulation.

Nutrition (per serving) Calories: 220; Total Fat: 4g; Saturated Fat: 0g; Cholesterol: 0mg; Sodium: 11mg; Potassium: 488mg; Magnesium: 84mg; Total Carbohydrates: 40g; Fiber: 9g; Sugars: 1g; Protein: 10g

VEGAN 30-MIN $-SAVER

White Bean and Roasted Red Pepper Soup

SERVES 4 • PREP TIME: 10 MINUTES • COOK TIME: 45 MINUTES

This delicious white-bean soup is made flavorful with red peppers, which are roasted in the oven before adding to the soup. Simple to prepare, this healthy and nutritious soup is high in the antioxidant vitamin C, potassium, protein, and fiber. Serve with crusty whole-grain bread.

3 large red bell peppers

1 tablespoon olive oil

1 small onion, chopped

⅛ teaspoon crushed red pepper

2 cups low-sodium vegetable broth

2 cups water

1 (15-ounce) can cannellini (white kidney) beans, drained and rinsed

1. Preheat the broiler to high. Place the bell peppers on a baking sheet. Broil, turning peppers frequently, until sides are blistered and charred. Remove from broiler.

2. Carefully place peppers in a plastic or paper bag; let stand 20 minutes. Peel off the layer of skin, and remove core and seeds.

3. Heat the olive oil in a large skillet over medium-high heat. Add the onion. Cook, stirring occasionally, for 3 to 5 minutes, or until the onions are tender.

4. Add the roasted peppers and crushed red pepper and cook for 1 minute.

5. Stir in the broth, water, and beans. Bring to a boil. Reduce the heat to low, and cook for 5 minutes.

6. Serve immediately.

INGREDIENT TIP Canned and jarred roasted red peppers tend to be very high in sodium. If you choose to use the canned or jarred variety to save time, be certain to rinse them in a colander to remove as much of the sodium as possible.

Nutrition (per serving) Calories: 169; Total Fat: 5g; Saturated Fat: 1g; Cholesterol: 0mg; Sodium: 180mg; Potassium: 196mg; Magnesium: 66mg; Total Carbohydrates: 26g; Fiber: 8g; Sugars: 4g; Protein: 7g

Tomato-Avocado Soup

SERVES 4 • PREP TIME: 5 MINUTES • COOK TIME: 12 MINUTES

Incredibly nutritious, half of an avocado contains 658 mg of potassium, 7 g of cholesterol-lowering fiber, and oleic acid, which reduces inflammation in the body. Low-fat buttermilk is used in place of heavy cream in this recipe, creating a rich and hearty soup that's perfect for a chilly afternoon.

½ tablespoon olive oil

1 cup chopped onion

1 clove garlic, minced

1 (14.5-ounce) can no-salt diced tomatoes in juice

1 cup low-sodium vegetable broth

1 cup water

½ teaspoon freshly ground black pepper

1 cup low-fat buttermilk

1 large ripe avocado, halved, pitted, peeled, and sliced

1. Heat the olive oil in a large pot over medium heat. Add the onion, and cook, stirring frequently, about 5 minutes, or until translucent. Add the garlic, and cook for 1 minute.

2. Transfer the onion-and-garlic mixture to a blender. Add the tomatoes and their juice, broth, water, and black pepper, and purée until smooth.

3. Transfer the purée back to the pot and heat the soup mixture over medium-low heat for 5 minutes, or until heated through. Add the buttermilk, and stir to combine.

4. Garnish each serving with a quarter of the avocado slices.

INGREDIENT TIP Low-fat buttermilk adds calcium and protein to this recipe along with beneficial probiotic bacteria, which aid in the absorption and digestion of some nutrients in the digestive tract.

Nutrition (per serving) Calories: 155; Total Fat: 9g; Saturated Fat: 2g; Cholesterol: 3mg; Sodium: 116mg; Potassium: 653mg; Magnesium: 40mg; Total Carbohydrates: 17g; Fiber: 5g; Sugars: 4g; Protein: 5g

Red Lentil Stew

SERVES 4 • PREP TIME: 5 MINUTES • COOK TIME: 40 MINUTES

Lentils are one of the most nutritious foods you can include in your diet. A type of legume, lentils are lower in calories and higher in protein and fiber than beans. Lentils contain a type of soluble fiber shown to reduce cholesterol, and they are a rich source of folate and magnesium, two nutrients that can reduce your risk for heart disease. These benefits make this lentil stew a comfort food that also follows the DASH-diet guidelines.

1 yellow onion, chopped

2 garlic cloves, minced

1 small bell pepper, chopped

3 medium carrots, peeled and chopped

1 (14.5-ounce) can no-salt diced tomatoes in juice

1 cup dried red lentils, rinsed

5 cups low-sodium vegetable broth

1. Spray a large pot with nonstick cooking spray and heat over medium heat. Add the onions and garlic and sauté until translucent, about 5 minutes.

2. Add the pepper and carrots, and sauté for 2 to 3 minutes.

3. Add the tomatoes and their juice, lentils, and vegetable broth and bring to a boil.

4. Reduce the heat to low. Cover the pot and simmer for about 30 minutes, until the lentils are tender.

5. Ladle the stew into soup bowls and serve.

INGREDIENT TIP Add 2 to 3 handfuls of spinach at the end of cooking for added calcium, magnesium, and potassium. A handful of fresh basil rounds out the flavor profile as well.

Nutrition (per serving) Calories: 197; Total Fat: 1g; Saturated Fat: 0g; Cholesterol: 0mg; Sodium: 222mg; Potassium: 889mg; Magnesium: 64mg; Total Carbohydrates: 38g; Fiber: 13g; Sugars: 6g; Protein: 11g

Pasta Primavera

SERVES 4 • PREP TIME: 10 MINUTES • COOK TIME: 15 MINUTES

Traditional pasta primavera uses a heavy cream sauce. This lighter DASH version is much lower in calories, fat, and sodium, and higher in fiber with a fresher taste. With several servings of vegetables, a serving of dairy, and a serving of whole grains, this is a healthy, delicious meal you can feel good about eating.

2 cups broccoli florets

1 cup sliced mushrooms

1 cup sliced zucchini or yellow squash

1 tablespoon olive oil, plus 1 teaspoon

2 garlic cloves, minced

¾ cup fat-free evaporated milk

½ cup freshly grated Parmesan cheese

8 ounces whole-wheat angel-hair or spaghetti pasta

⅓ cup chopped fresh parsley (optional)

1. In a large pot fitted with a steamer basket, bring about 1 inch of water to a boil. Add the broccoli, mushrooms, and zucchini. Cover and steam until tender-crisp, about 10 minutes. Remove from the pot.

2. In a large saucepan, heat 1 tablespoon of the olive oil over medium heat. Add the garlic and sauté over medium heat for 2 to 3 minutes. Add the steamed vegetables and stir or shake to coat the vegetables with the garlic. Remove the saucepan from the heat but keep warm.

3. In another large saucepan, heat the remaining 1 teaspoon of olive oil, evaporated milk, and Parmesan cheese. Stir continuously over medium heat until somewhat thickened and heated through without scalding. Remove the saucepan from the heat but keep warm.

continued >

4. Fill a large pot three-quarters full with water and bring to a boil. Add the pasta and cook according to the package directions, until the desired doneness. Drain the pasta.

5. Divide the pasta evenly among four plates. Top each serving with a quarter of the vegetables and Parmesan sauce. Garnish with fresh parsley (if using) and serve immediately.

BUDGET-SAVER TIP You can use frozen vegetables in place of the fresh to keep costs in check and cut down on prep time. A 16-ounce bag of frozen vegetables is equivalent to about 2 cups fresh.

Nutrition (per serving) Calories: 350; Total Fat: 9g; Saturated Fat: 3g; Cholesterol: 12mg; Sodium: 317mg; Potassium: 491mg; Magnesium: 44mg; Total Carbohydrates: 53g; Fiber: 7g; Sugars: 7g; Protein: 17g

Penne with White Beans and Roasted Tomato Sauce

SERVES 4 • PREP TIME: 5 MINUTES • COOK TIME: 25 MINUTES

This high-fiber, low-sodium, nutrient-rich penne recipe gets its rich taste from fresh cherry tomatoes, which are lightly roasted in the oven. Full of plant-powered protein and potassium from white beans, be certain to choose whole-wheat penne for the most health benefits.

2 pints cherry tomatoes, halved

2 tablespoons chopped fresh basil

2 tablespoons olive oil, divided

8 ounces whole-wheat penne

2 garlic cloves, minced

1 (15-ounce) can white beans (navy or great northern), drained and rinsed

1 tablespoon balsamic vinegar

1. Preheat the oven to 425°F.

2. On a large sheet pan, toss the tomatoes with the basil and 1 tablespoon of the olive oil. Place the pan in the oven and roast until wilted and beginning to brown, about 20 minutes.

3. Meanwhile, cook the penne according to the package directions. Reserve ¼ cup of the cooking water, and drain. Add the pasta, beans, tomato mixture, garlic, balsamic vinegar, and the cooking water to a medium pot and simmer for 2 minutes.

4. Drizzle the pasta with the remaining 1 tablespoon of olive oil and serve.

INGREDIENT TIP If you're not a fan of whole-wheat pasta, there are a number of alternatives available. Most grocery stores now carry pastas made from lentils, black beans, and quinoa, which add more protein and fiber.

Nutrition (per serving) Calories: 370; Total Fat: 9g; Saturated Fat: 1g; Cholesterol: 0mg; Sodium: 121mg; Potassium: 317mg; Magnesium: 36mg; Total Carbohydrates: 66g; Fiber: 6g; Sugars: 1g; Protein: 13g

Chickpea Burgers

SERVES 4 • PREP TIME: 5 MINUTES • COOK TIME: 30 MINUTES

Delicious and hearty, these chickpea burgers can be made quickly using whole-food ingredients that contribute to heart health and healthy blood pressure. With healthy fats from walnuts, soluble fiber from oats, and protein and potassium from beans, you'll love these burgers topped with your favorite burger fixings.

2 teaspoons olive oil

1 small yellow onion, diced

2 cups rolled oats (not instant)

½ cup ground walnuts

1 (15-ounce) can chickpeas, drained and rinsed

¾ cup nonfat or low-fat milk

½ teaspoon garlic powder

½ teaspoon onion powder

½ teaspoon dried sage

1. In a large skillet, heat the olive oil. Add the onions and cook for about 10 minutes, until very tender and golden brown. Set aside.

2. In a large bowl, toss together the oats and ground walnuts. Set aside.

3. In a blender, combine the chickpeas, milk, garlic powder, onion powder, and dried sage, and process until smooth and creamy.

4. Pour the chickpea mixture into the bowl with the oats and walnuts. Add the browned onions and mix well.

5. Allow the mixture to rest for 5 to 10 minutes, so the oats can absorb the liquid.

6. Form the mixture into eight thin, flat patties. Using the same skillet, brown the burgers over medium-low heat for 5 to 7 minutes on each side.

7. Serve with your favorite toppings.

INGREDIENT TIP These burgers freeze well by wrapping them individually in plastic wrap and covering with foil. Make a double batch on the weekend and freeze a batch so you have a healthy meal in your freezer for those busy nights.

Nutrition (per serving) Calories: 375; Total Fat: 16g; Saturated Fat: 1g; Cholesterol: 1mg; Sodium: 112mg; Potassium: 172mg; Magnesium: 40mg; Total Carbohydrates: 48g; Fiber: 11g; Sugars: 4g; Protein: 14g

Tofu Scramble with Potatoes and Mushrooms

SERVES 4 • PREP TIME: 10 MINUTES • COOK TIME: 15 MINUTES

Tofu can easily be transformed into "mock" scrambled eggs that rival their egg counterpart in taste, but come with none of the cholesterol or saturated fat. Paired with potassium-rich potatoes, this tofu scramble is filling, flavorful, and full of blood pressure–lowering nutrients.

1 large Yukon gold potato, peeled and cut into ½-inch pieces

1 tablespoon olive oil

1 bunch scallions, thinly sliced

2 garlic cloves

1 teaspoon chili powder

1 teaspoon cumin

2 cups sliced mushrooms

1 (14-ounce) block firm tofu, drained and crumbled

1 large tomato, sliced or diced (optional)

1. Place the potato pieces in a large skillet and cover with water. Bring to a boil, then reduce the heat to medium and simmer for 3 minutes. Pour out all but 1 tablespoon of the water.

2. Add the olive oil, scallions, garlic, chili powder, and cumin to the skillet, and cook, stirring, for 2 minutes. Add the mushrooms and cook, stirring occasionally, for 5 to 7 minutes, or until the potatoes are tender and mushrooms are browned.

3. Add the tofu and 2 tablespoons of cooking water and cook until the tofu is heated through, about 3 more minutes.

4. Divide the scramble among four plates and serve with tomato slices (if using).

INGREDIENT TIP You can boost the fiber and minerals in this recipe by adding a bunch of spinach when the tofu is added. This will add more calcium, magnesium, and potassium to the dish. Feel free to customize with your favorite fresh or frozen veggies.

Nutrition (per serving) Calories: 186; Total Fat: 10g; Saturated Fat: 2g; Cholesterol: 0mg; Sodium: 33mg; Potassium: 672mg; Magnesium: 104mg; Total Carbohydrates: 14g; Fiber: 4g; Sugars: 3g; Protein: 15g

Mexican Beans and Rice

SERVES 4 • PREP TIME: 5 MINUTES • COOK TIME: 35 MINUTES

If you have been looking for the perfect Mexican rice recipe, then look no further! Easy and delicious, this fiber-rich dish uses medium-grain rice, which yields a tender, starchy, slightly creamy kernel that's ideal for saucy rice dishes like this. With ample plant protein from black beans, this dish also makes a great accompaniment to pork tenderloin.

1 cup uncooked medium-grain brown rice

2 cups cold water

1 (14.5 ounce) can no-salt diced tomatoes in juice

2 tablespoons olive oil

6 garlic cloves, finely chopped

1 medium jalapeño pepper, cored, seeded, and finely chopped

1 (15-ounce) can black beans, drained and rinsed

2 teaspoons cumin

1 teaspoon chili powder

¼ cup finely chopped fresh oregano

¼ cup finely chopped fresh cilantro

1. In a 1-quart saucepan, combine the rice with the cold water. Bring to a boil over medium-high heat. Cover, reduce heat to low, and simmer for 20 minutes.

2. Remove the pan from the heat and let stand, covered, another 5 minutes.

3. While the rice steams, set a fine colander or sieve in a bowl and drain the can of tomatoes. Pour the tomato juices into a 1-cup liquid measure. Add enough water to the tomato juice to equal 1 cup. Set the tomatoes aside.

4. Heat the olive oil in a medium skillet over medium-high heat. Add the garlic and jalapeño, and stir-fry until the garlic browns and the jalapeño smells pungent, about 1 minute.

5. Add the black beans, cumin, and chili powder; stir two to three times to incorporate the mixture and cook the spices, about 30 seconds.

continued >

6. Stir in the tomato liquid and bring to a boil. Adjust the heat to maintain a gentle boil and cook, stirring occasionally, for 5 to 7 minutes, or until the beans absorb much of the liquid.

7. Add the tomatoes, oregano, cilantro, and cooked rice. Continue cooking, stirring occasionally, for 1 to 2 minutes, or until the rice is warm.

8. Serve immediately.

BUDGET-SAVER TIP You can substitute dried herbs in place of the fresh herbs to keep your costs in check. Because dried herbs are more potent than fresh, you'll need less. Use 1 tablespoon of the dried variety in place of ¼ cup of the fresh.

Nutrition (per serving) Calories: 356; Total Fat: 10g; Saturated Fat: 1g; Cholesterol: 0mg; Sodium: 128mg; Potassium: 439mg; Magnesium: 53mg; Total Carbohydrates: 59g; Fiber: 11g; Sugars: 0g; Protein: 11g

Sweet Potato and Black Bean Wraps

SERVES 4 • PREP TIME: 10 MINUTES • COOK TIME: 20 MINUTES

Rich in potassium, magnesium, fiber, and vitamin A, sweet potatoes are combined with equally nutritious black beans in this quick-to-prepare, delicious dish. For a lower-calorie recipe, use romaine lettuce leaves in place of the corn tortillas.

1 large sweet potato, cubed

2 teaspoons olive oil

½ small onion, finely chopped

1 bell pepper, chopped

2 garlic cloves, minced

2 teaspoons cumin

1 (15-ounce) can black beans, drained and rinsed

1 cup cooked brown rice

8 small corn tortillas

TOPPINGS

1 to 2 slices avocado (optional)

1 to 2 slices tomato (optional)

¼ cup shredded lettuce (optional)

2 tablespoons chopped fresh cilantro (optional)

1. Preheat the oven to 425°F and line a baking sheet with foil. Spread the sweet potato evenly over the baking sheet, spray with nonstick cooking spray, and roast for 15 to 20 minutes, or until tender.

2. Meanwhile, in a large skillet over medium heat, add the olive oil, onion, bell pepper, and minced garlic. Sauté for 5 to 10 minutes, stirring frequently. Add the cumin and stir well.

3. Add the beans and cooked rice, and sauté for another 5 minutes over medium heat.

4. Add the roasted sweet potato to the rice mixture and stir well, mashing some of the larger pieces of sweet potato if desired.

5. Add the filling to the tortillas along with your desired toppings, and serve immediately.

SUBSTITUTION TIP You can replace the rice with an additional cup of vegetables for fewer calories and carbohydrates and more nutrients and fiber. Some suggestions include 1 cup of broccoli florets, 1 cup of cauliflower florets, or 1 cup of finely shredded cabbage.

Nutrition (per serving) Calories: 301; Total Fat: 6g; Saturated Fat: 0g; Cholesterol: 0mg; Sodium: 157mg; Potassium: 214mg; Magnesium: 39mg; Total Carbohydrates: 55g; Fiber: 9g; Sugars: 1g; Protein: 11g

Spiced Lentils and Poached Eggs

SERVES 4 • PREP TIME: 10 MINUTES • COOK TIME: 35 MINUTES

This delicious, flavorful, and satisfying recipe may just become one of your go-to recipes when you want a healthy and balanced meal fast. Fragrant Indian spices give this dish a bit of heat, which is tempered with a dollop of calcium-rich Greek yogurt on top. Full of fiber, protein, magnesium, and calcium, this dish pairs nicely with a spinach salad to complete your DASH dinner.

1 cup dried small red lentils

3 cups water

1 bay leaf

2 teaspoons olive oil

1 cup chopped onion

1 cup chopped tomato

1 teaspoon curry powder

¼ teaspoon ground cumin

2 garlic cloves, minced

1 tablespoon white vinegar

4 large eggs

¼ teaspoon freshly ground black pepper

¼ cup low-fat plain Greek yogurt, divided

¼ cup chopped fresh cilantro, for garnish (optional)

1. Combine the lentils, water, and bay leaf in a large saucepan. Bring to a boil. Cover, reduce the heat, and simmer for 20 minutes or until lentils are tender. Drain, and discard the bay leaf.

2. Heat a nonstick skillet over medium-high heat. Add the olive oil to the pan and swirl to coat. Add the onion and tomato and sauté for 8 minutes, or until the onion is tender. Add the curry, cumin, and garlic, and sauté for 2 minutes. Add the lentils, and cook for 1 minute. Remove the skillet from the heat.

3. Add enough water to a large skillet to fill it two-thirds full. Bring the water to a boil, and then reduce the heat to simmer. Add the white vinegar to the water.

4. Break the eggs, one at a time, into a custard cup, and gently pour into the water. Poach the eggs for 3 minutes or until your desired doneness. Using a slotted spoon, carefully remove eggs from the skillet.

5. Divide the lentil mixture among four serving plates and top each serving with 1 poached egg. Sprinkle evenly with the black pepper and top each serving with 1 tablespoon of the yogurt and 1 tablespoon of the cilantro (if using).

INGREDIENT TIP Lentils are marketed in four general categories: brown, green, red/yellow, and specialty, and within each category are several varieties, which makes for fun discovery and experimentation. In general, the brown and green varieties hold their shape well, while red tend to disintegrate, and specialty fall somewhere in between.

Nutrition (per serving) Calories: 213; Total Fat: 8g; Saturated Fat: 2g; Cholesterol: 188mg; Sodium: 86mg; Potassium: 566mg; Magnesium: 48mg; Total Carbohydrates: 28g; Fiber: 13g; Sugars: 3g; Protein: 19g

Asparagus and Mushroom Crustless Quiche

SERVES 4 • PREP TIME: 5 MINUTES • COOK TIME: 45 MINUTES

This crustless quiche is a great way to incorporate more vegetables into your diet without any fuss. This version uses asparagus, a natural diuretic, and mushrooms, which are rich in vitamin D, but you can add in any of your other favorite vegetables. Caramelizing the onions first gives the quiche a little sweetness, and it's great served warm or at room temperature.

1 tablespoon olive oil

1 large yellow or white onion, sliced into half-moons

½ teaspoon freshly ground black pepper

2 cups chopped mushrooms

2 cups chopped asparagus

4 large eggs

4 large egg whites

1 cup nonfat or low-fat milk

½ cup shredded low-fat cheese

1. Preheat the oven to 350°F.

2. Heat the olive oil in a cast iron or ovenproof skillet over medium heat. Add the onion slices and sprinkle with the black pepper. Cook the onions until they are golden brown and starting to caramelize, about 10 minutes.

3. Remove the skillet from the heat and spread the onions evenly across the bottom. Spread the mushrooms and asparagus evenly over the onions.

4. In a medium bowl, add the eggs, egg whites, milk, cheese, and black pepper. Stir with a fork, beating just enough to break up the yolks and white. Pour the custard over the vegetables and onions.

5. Transfer the skillet to the oven, and bake for 45 minutes to 1 hour, until fully cooked and lightly browned across the top. Let the quiche cool for 20 minutes, and then slice into four wedges.

SUBSTITUTION TIP If you decide to use hardier vegetables like broccoli, cauliflower, or winter squash, be sure to cook them before adding them to the skillet to ensure they'll be tender when served. Quick-cooking vegetables can be used fresh.

Nutrition (per serving) Calories: 213; Total Fat: 11g; Saturated Fat: 3g; Cholesterol: 195mg; Sodium: 256mg; Potassium: 520mg; Magnesium: 28mg; Total Carbohydrates: 12g; Fiber: 3g; Sugars: 4g; Protein: 19g

Egg-Topped Rice Bowl

SERVES 2 • PREP TIME: 5 MINUTES • COOK TIME: 10 MINUTES

This super-easy recipe is a bowl of fiber-rich rice and veggies with a twist. Here, the yolk of the fried egg serves as a dressing to coat the rice without having to do anything extra. Spinach adds valuable amounts of calcium, magnesium, and potassium, which are important for blood-pressure regulation and also aid in the absorption of the vitamin D in the egg yolk. A dash of hot sauce gives this dish a bit of a kick.

1 bunch spinach
(about 5 ounces)

½ cup halved
cherry tomatoes

1 teaspoon red
wine vinegar

1 cup cooked
brown rice, warm

⅓ cup sliced avocado

1 teaspoon olive oil

2 large eggs

⅛ teaspoon freshly
ground black pepper

½ teaspoon hot sauce
(optional)

1. Heat a large nonstick skillet over medium heat. Add the spinach and cook for 2 minutes, or until the spinach wilts. Stir in the tomatoes and red wine vinegar, and remove the skillet from the heat.

2. Divide the rice evenly between two bowls and top evenly with the spinach mixture. Arrange the avocado slices alongside the spinach mixture.

3. Wipe the skillet dry with a paper towel, and return it to medium heat. Add the olive oil to the skillet and swirl to coat. Crack the eggs, one at a time, into the skillet. Cook the eggs for 2 minutes, and then cover and cook for 1 minute, or until the whites are set.

4. Top each bowl of rice with the cooked egg. Sprinkle evenly with the black pepper and hot sauce (if using). Serve immediately.

INGREDIENT TIP For added nutrition, consider using omega-3 eggs, which are produced by hens that are fed flaxseeds. These eggs contain significant levels of omega-3 fatty acids, which are not only heart-healthy but also have been shown to reduce inflammation in the body. They cost only slightly more than regular eggs, but the added health benefits may be worth it.

Nutrition (per serving) Calories: 312; Total Fat: 15g; Saturated Fat: 3g; Cholesterol: 186mg; Sodium: 213mg; Potassium: 1,372mg; Magnesium: 192mg; Total Carbohydrates: 35g; Fiber: 9g; Sugars: 1g; Protein: 15g

Asparagus and Wild Garlic Risotto

SERVES 4 • PREP TIME: 10 MINUTES • COOK TIME: 40 MINUTES

Risotto is a creamy rice dish that typically uses butter, cheese, and some type of broth. The dish has a reputation for being complicated to cook, however, you can easily make your own risotto at home and be pleased with the results. This recipe includes vitamin- and mineral-rich asparagus and lightens things up by making it dairy-free. This creamy, delicious dish is healthy and perfect for spring. The slow method of cooking the rice ensures that the starch is released from the rice for the creamy texture risotto is known for.

8 cups no-salt vegetable broth

2 tablespoons olive oil

4 garlic cloves, minced

1 cup Arborio rice

1 cup white wine

Zest and juice of 1 lemon

1 bunch asparagus, trimmed and thinly sliced

¼ chopped fresh sage

1. In a large pot, bring the broth just to a simmer.

2. Meanwhile, heat a large skillet over medium heat. Add the olive oil and heat for 30 to 60 seconds, until shimmering. Add the garlic and cook for 30 seconds.

3. Add the rice. Cook, stirring constantly for about 1 minute, and then add the wine. Continue to stir and cook, allowing the wine to absorb into the rice. Add the lemon zest and juice, and stir.

4. Reduce the heat to medium-low, and ladle about 1 cup of the warm broth into the skillet. Cook, stirring constantly, allowing the liquid to be absorbed completely.

5. Add another cup of broth and continue to stir, once again allowing the liquid to be absorbed completely. Repeat with additional broth until the rice is creamy and cooked through for an al dente (or slightly firm) consistency.

6. Remove the skillet from the heat, and stir in the uncooked asparagus and sage. Serve immediately.

SUBSTITUTION TIP If you want to make a more traditional risotto, add 1 to 2 tablespoons of margarine and ½ to ¾ cup of finely grated, low-fat Parmigiano-Reggiano cheese right before you add the asparagus.

Nutrition (per serving) Calories: 288; Total Fat: 7g; Saturated Fat: 1g; Cholesterol: 0mg; Sodium: 6mg; Potassium: 332mg; Magnesium: 24mg; Total Carbohydrates: 42g; Fiber: 3g; Sugars: 0g; Protein: 6g

Enchiladas with Bean Medley

SERVES 4 • PREP TIME: 15 MINUTES • COOK TIME: 35 MINUTES

This delicious vegetarian enchilada recipe is full of plant-powered protein and blood pressure–lowering minerals. With black beans, green beans, and low-fat cheese, this vegetarian entrée is balanced in nutrition and food-group servings.

2 tablespoons olive oil

1 pound green beans, washed and ends snipped

1 teaspoon cumin

1 (15-ounce) can black beans, drained and rinsed

1 cup shredded low-fat Monterey Jack cheese, divided

1 (14-ounce) can red enchilada sauce

Freshly ground black pepper

8 corn tortillas

1. Preheat the oven to 400°F with one rack in the middle of the oven and one in the upper third. Lightly grease a 9-by-13-inch baking pan with nonstick cooking spray.

2. In a large skillet over medium heat, heat the olive oil until shimmering. Add the green beans and cook, stirring occasionally, for 5 to 7 minutes, or until the green beans are brighter green. Add the cumin to the skillet, and cook until fragrant, about 30 seconds.

3. Transfer the contents of the pan to a medium-size mixing bowl. Add the black beans, ¼ cup of the cheese, and about 2 tablespoons of the enchilada sauce. Season with black pepper.

4. Assemble the enchiladas: Pour ¼ cup of the enchilada sauce into the prepared pan and tilt it from side to side until the bottom of the pan is evenly coated.

5. To assemble the enchiladas, spread ¼ cup of the filling mixture down the middle of a tortilla, and then snugly wrap the left side over and then the right to make a wrap. Place it in the pan and repeat with the remaining tortillas and filling.

6. Drizzle the remaining enchilada sauce evenly over the enchiladas, leaving the ends of the enchiladas bare. Sprinkle the remaining cheese evenly over the enchiladas.

7. Bake, uncovered, on the middle rack, for 20 minutes. If the cheese isn't golden enough to your liking, carefully transfer the enchiladas to the upper rack and bake for an additional 3 to 6 minutes, or until golden and bubbly.

8. Serve immediately.

SUBSTITUTION TIP You can make this recipe vegan by omitting the cheese altogether and topping with sliced avocado for some extra creaminess.

Nutrition (per serving) Calories: 368; Total Fat: 18g; Saturated Fat: 1g; Cholesterol: 0mg; Sodium: 616mg; Potassium: 237mg; Magnesium: 39mg; Total Carbohydrates: 40g; Fiber: 11g; Sugars: 1g; Protein: 18g

Chicken Legs with
Rice and Peas,
page 103

CHAPTER 6

Poultry & Seafood Entrées

Spinach-Stuffed Turkey Burgers

SERVES 4 • PREP TIME: 15 MINUTES • COOK TIME: 15 MINUTES

This recipe starts as a burger, but with the addition of fresh baby spinach, it becomes a vegetable lover's delight that is perfect for the DASH eating plan. High-fiber and cholesterol-lowering oats are incorporated into the patties to give them a great texture, and garlic and lemon provide a just-right taste. Serve this burger with your favorite toppings on a whole-grain bun.

12 ounces 93% lean ground turkey

4 cups fresh baby spinach

⅓ cup rolled oats

2 garlic cloves, minced

1 egg, beaten

2 teaspoons freshly squeezed lemon juice

¾ teaspoon freshly ground black pepper

1 teaspoon hot sauce (optional)

1. In a medium bowl, combine all of the ingredients, and mix until well incorporated. Using your hands, form the mixture into four 5-inch-wide patties.

2. Spray a large skillet with nonstick cooking spray, and place it over medium heat. Place the patties in the skillet and cook for 7 to 8 minutes on each side, or until well done and browned and an instant-read thermometer registers 165°F.

3. Serve with your favorite toppings.

INGREDIENT TIP You can boost the veggie content further by adding ½ cup of shredded carrots or shredded zucchini to the mixture. You can also add ¼ cup chopped fresh cilantro for a flavor boost.

Nutrition (per serving) Calories: 173; Total Fat: 8g; Saturated Fat: 2g; Cholesterol: 107mg; Sodium: 106mg; Potassium: 196mg; Magnesium: 24mg; Total Carbohydrates: 6g; Fiber: 2g; Sugars: 0g; Protein: 20g

Ground Turkey–Brussels Sprouts Skillet

SERVES 4 • PREP TIME: 10 MINUTES • COOK TIME: 30 MINUTES

This nutritious one-pot skillet dish combines lean ground turkey, Brussels sprouts, peppers, and spices for a delicious balanced meal that follows the DASH guidelines. Brussels sprouts and peppers are rich in the antioxidant vitamin C, fiber, and important phytochemicals that can reduce inflammation in the body. Choose lean ground turkey to keep unhealthy fats in check.

2 tablespoons olive oil, divided

1 red onion, diced

1 pound 93% lean ground turkey

4 garlic cloves, minced

2 teaspoons chili powder

½ pound Brussels sprouts, shredded

1 bell pepper, diced

1. In a large skillet over medium heat, warm 1 tablespoon of the olive oil. Add the onion and stir-fry for 5 minutes, or until the onion is soft.

2. Add the ground turkey, garlic, and chili powder, and cook, stirring occasionally, for 15 to 20 minutes, until the meat is completely cooked through and no longer pink, and an instant-read thermometer registers 165°F.

3. Set aside some of the turkey in a bowl to make room for the Brussels sprouts and bell pepper. Add the remaining 1 tablespoon of oil to the skillet, and add the Brussels sprouts and bell pepper. Stir-fry for 5 minutes, or until the vegetables are tender.

4. Add the meat back to the pan and mix well. Serve immediately.

Nutrition (per serving) Calories: 262; Total Fat: 16g; Saturated Fat: 4g; Cholesterol: 80mg; Sodium: 114mg; Potassium: 314mg; Magnesium: 20mg; Total Carbohydrates: 9g; Fiber: 3g; Sugars: 3g; Protein: 25g

Chicken Salad with Creamy Tarragon Dressing

SERVES 4 • PREP TIME: 15 MINUTES • COOK TIME: 5 MINUTES

If you have been avoiding chicken salad, which tends to be very high in sodium, calories, and unhealthy fats, then this recipe will satisfy your taste buds while still fitting into the DASH eating plan. The trick is in the healthy salad dressing, which is made using beans, olive oil, and vinegar, instead of fatty mayonnaise. Full of high-quality lean protein, fiber, vitamins, and minerals, this dish is very quick to prepare.

1 (15-ounce) can white beans, drained and rinsed, divided

⅓ cup white balsamic vinegar

1 tablespoon olive oil

2 garlic cloves

2 teaspoons dried tarragon, divided

6 cups salad greens

½ red onion, thinly sliced

1½ cups chopped cooked chicken breast

1 cup English cucumber, thinly sliced

¾ teaspoon freshly ground black pepper

1. In a blender, combine ½ cup of the beans, the balsamic vinegar, olive oil, garlic, and 1 teaspoon of tarragon, and purée.

2. Arrange the greens on four serving plates. Top with the remaining beans, onion, chicken, cucumber, black pepper, and remaining tarragon.

3. Serve the dressing on the side.

INGREDIENT TIP Roast a few boneless, skinless chicken breasts and keep them in the refrigerator for recipes that call for precooked chicken such as this one. Alternatively, you could pick up a rotisserie chicken, but be sure to remove the skin and use the white meat only. Some rotisserie chickens are high in sodium so check the nutrition facts panel before purchasing.

Nutrition (per serving) Calories: 267; Total Fat: 7g; Saturated Fat: 1g; Cholesterol: 53mg; Sodium: 196mg; Potassium: 484mg; Magnesium: 49mg; Total Carbohydrates: 25g; Fiber: 8g; Sugars: 1g; Protein: 28g

Tandoori Chicken with Rice

SERVES 4 • PREP TIME: 20 MINUTES • COOK TIME: 30 MINUTES

Skip the takeout and make your own much-healthier version of this popular dish from India. This recipe for Tandoori chicken is spice-filled and offers a lot of flavor without the use of salt or unhealthy fats. A side dish of steamed green peas finishes off this meal.

1 pound boneless, skinless chicken breast or tenderloins, trimmed of visible fat

¼ cup lemon juice

½ cup plain nonfat Greek yogurt

3 garlic cloves, minced

1 teaspoon curry powder

1 teaspoon ground ginger

1 teaspoon paprika

1 teaspoon ground cumin

1 cup instant brown rice

1. Preheat the oven to 400°F.

2. Place the chicken in a 9-by-9-inch baking dish and pierce the chicken pieces all over with a fork.

3. In a small bowl, whisk together the lemon juice, Greek yogurt, garlic, curry powder, ginger, paprika, and cumin. Pour the spice mixture over the chicken, turning to coat. Let stand for 20 minutes.

4. Place the chicken in the oven and bake for 15 minutes. Turn the chicken, and bake for 15 minutes more, or until an instant-read thermometer registers 165°F.

5. While the chicken bakes, prepare the rice according to the package directions.

6. Divide the rice among four plates, and top each serving with chicken. Serve immediately.

BUDGET-SAVER TIP Green peas are traditionally served with Tandoori chicken. Frozen green peas are your healthiest bet and are readily available and economical. Keep a bag or two on hand in the freezer for a healthy and nutritious side dish.

Nutrition (per serving) Calories: 246; Total Fat: 5g; Saturated Fat: 2g; Cholesterol: 66mg; Sodium: 61mg; Potassium: 157mg; Magnesium: 36mg; Total Carbohydrates: 22g; Fiber: 2g; Sugars: 2g; Protein: 30g

Apricot Chicken

SERVES 4 • PREP TIME: 5 MINUTES • COOK TIME: 30 MINUTES

One of the most versatile and low-calorie fruits, apricots are extremely nutritious and DASH-friendly. This little orange fruit boasts high levels of potassium, vitamin A, vitamin C, and fiber. Apricots can be eaten in multiple ways, working equally well in sweet dishes like your morning oats, or savory dishes like this quick-and-easy chicken entrée. Serve with a side of steamed broccoli.

2 teaspoons olive oil

1 pound boneless, skinless chicken breasts, trimmed and cut into 4 pieces

8 to 9 ripe apricots, pitted and chopped

½ cup dry white wine

½ cup no-salt chicken stock

Juice of 1 orange

¼ cup honey

1 teaspoon dried thyme

1 tablespoon fresh orange zest

1. Heat a large nonstick skillet over medium-high heat, and heat the olive oil. Place the chicken breasts in the pan and cook for 5 to 8 minutes per side, or until an instant-read thermometer registers 165°F. Transfer the chicken breasts to a clean plate and cover with foil to keep warm.

2. In the same skillet, add the apricots, wine, chicken stock, orange juice, and honey. Turn the heat to high and allow the liquid to come to a boil. Boil, uncovered, for about 10 minutes, stirring occasionally. The liquid should reduce by half, and the apricots should break down a little but still be somewhat chunky. The sauce should be on the thick side.

3. Remove the sauce from the heat and stir in the thyme and orange zest. Spoon the sauce over the warm chicken breasts.

4. Serve immediately with a desired side dish.

INGREDIENT TIP For a roasted broccoli side dish, preheat the oven to 400°F. Arrange the broccoli florets on a large rimmed baking sheet. Toss with 2 teaspoons of olive oil and season with black pepper. Roast for 25 to 30 minutes, flipping halfway through. The small bits should be slightly charred and crispy.

Nutrition (per serving) Calories: 287; Total Fat: 7g; Saturated Fat: 2g; Cholesterol: 65mg; Sodium: 49mg; Potassium: 256mg; Magnesium: 12mg; Total Carbohydrates: 28g; Fiber: 2g; Sugars: 25g; Protein: 27g

Pistachio-Crusted Chicken

SERVES 4 • PREP TIME: 10 MINUTES • COOK TIME: 30 MINUTES

If you haven't added pistachios to your snacking routine yet, then you are missing out. You can eat more pistachios per serving than any other kind of nut. A serving of 30 pistachios is the perfect 100-calorie snack. Plus, pistachios are very heart-healthy with their good-for-you fats, high levels of vitamin E, a type of fiber shown to reduce cholesterol, high levels of potassium, and plant antioxidants that can reduce inflammation. The perfect nut to cook with, pistachios are used as the crust in this easy chicken recipe.

½ cup finely chopped pistachio nuts (shelled)

½ teaspoon freshly ground black pepper

1 pound boneless, skinless chicken breasts, trimmed and cut into 4 pieces

2 tablespoons olive oil

1. Preheat the oven to 350°F.

2. In a small bowl or bag, combine the pistachio nuts and black pepper.

3. Brush the chicken breasts with olive oil, then roll them in the bowl or shake them in the bag to cover both sides with the nut mixture.

4. Place the chicken breasts in a greased 9-by-13-inch pan. Bake for 25 to 35 minutes, or until juices run clear and an instant-read thermometer registers 165°F.

5. Serve immediately.

INGREDIENT TIP Pistachios can be stored in an airtight container in the refrigerator or freezer for maximum freshness. Airtight containers will keep your pistachios from absorbing moisture and going stale.

Nutrition (per serving) Calories: 286; Total Fat: 18g; Saturated Fat: 3g; Cholesterol: 65mg; Sodium: 40mg; Potassium: 3mg; Magnesium: 4mg; Total Carbohydrates: 5g; Fiber: 2g; Sugars: 1g; Protein: 28g

Shrimp and Avocado Salad

SERVES 4 • PREP TIME: 10 MINUTES

Serving an entrée salad is a great strategy for incorporating more servings of vegetables into your diet without a lot of fuss. This salad is perfect for a quick lunch or dinner, especially during the summer when you crave meals that are cool and filling without being heavy and draining. With healthy fats from creamy avocado and ample lean protein from shrimp, this salad also has some zest from the red onion and dressing.

1 pound cooked
salad shrimp

2 avocados, peeled,
pitted, and cubed

2 tomatoes, diced

2 tablespoons diced
red onion

8 cups fresh
baby spinach

FOR THE DRESSING

2 tablespoons olive oil

¼ cup red wine vinegar

1 teaspoon
parsley, chopped

1 teaspoon
Dijon mustard

½ teaspoon
garlic powder

1. In a large bowl, toss together the shrimp, avocados, tomatoes, and onion.

2. In a 2-cup measuring cup, mix together ingredients for the dressing. Whisk until well combined.

3. Pour the dressing over the shrimp to lightly coat as desired.

4. Divide the spinach among four serving plates, and top with the shrimp salad. Serve additional dressing on the side.

BUDGET-SAVER TIP Take advantage of your local farmers' markets during the summer to purchase fresh vegetables like tomatoes and spinach when they are less expensive.

Nutrition (per serving) Calories: 347; Total Fat: 21g; Saturated Fat: 3g; Cholesterol: 138mg; Sodium: 309mg; Potassium: 925mg; Magnesium: 80mg; Total Carbohydrates: 13g; Fiber: 9g; Sugars: 1g; Protein: 29g

Salmon and Asparagus in Foil

SERVES 4 • PREP TIME: 5 MINUTES • COOK TIME: 20 MINUTES

One of the best foods you can include in your DASH diet is fatty fish. The salmon you'll use in this dish is rich in omega-3 fatty acids, which reduce inflammation in the body, lower blood pressure, slow the growth rate of atherosclerotic plaque buildup, and lower triglyceride levels. With the added benefits of asparagus, a natural diuretic, this one-pan dish should become a regular part of your diet.

4 (5-ounce) salmon fillets

1 pound fresh asparagus, ends trimmed, divided

2 teaspoons dried dill, divided

Freshly squeezed lemon juice

Freshly ground black pepper (optional)

Lemon wedges for serving

1. Preheat the oven to 450°F.

2. Prepare four 12-by-18-inch sheets of aluminum foil. Spray the center of each sheet of foil with nonstick cooking spray.

3. Place one salmon fillet in the center of each sheet, top with a quarter of the asparagus, ½ teaspoon of dill, and a squeeze of lemon juice. Sprinkle with black pepper (if using).

4. Bring up the sides of the foil and fold the top over twice. Seal the ends, leaving room for air to circulate inside the packet. Repeat with the remaining fillets.

5. Place the packets on a baking sheet and bake for 15 to 18 minutes, or until the salmon is opaque.

6. Use caution when opening the packets, as the steam is very hot. Serve with lemon wedges on the side.

BUDGET-SAVER TIP Frozen salmon may be a better option for the budget-conscious. In terms of quality, most fish is flash-frozen when caught to preserve its freshness and allow for shipping.

Nutrition (per serving) Calories: 202; Total Fat: 7g; Saturated Fat: 1g; Cholesterol: 63mg; Sodium: 110mg; Potassium: 326mg; Magnesium: 24mg; Total Carbohydrates: 5g; Fiber: 3g; Sugars: 0g; Protein: 31g

Halibut with Greens and Ginger

SERVES 4 • PREP TIME: 5 MINUTES • COOK TIME: 10 MINUTES

Halibut is a type of fatty fish rich in heart-healthy omega-3 fatty acids, making it a great addition to your diet. While you may not consider fish to be rich sources of vitamins and minerals, a 6-ounce serving of halibut contains 40 percent of the RDA of magnesium, a mineral that's important for blood-pressure regulation. Used in this super-fast and easy recipe, halibut is paired with vitamin- and mineral-rich spinach to produce a very flavorful dish.

4 (4-ounce) halibut fillets, rinsed and patted dry

½ teaspoon freshly ground black pepper

3 teaspoons olive oil, divided

4 cups baby spinach

1 tablespoon minced peeled ginger

2 garlic cloves, minced

1 tablespoon balsamic vinegar

1 tablespoon freshly squeezed lime juice

1. Sprinkle the fish with the black pepper. Using your fingertips, gently press in the seasoning so it adheres to the fish.

2. In a large nonstick skillet, heat 2 teaspoons of the olive oil over medium-high heat, swirling to coat the bottom. Cook the fish for 2 minutes, or until browned on the bottom. Turn over, and cook for 2 minutes more, or until the fish flakes easily when tested with a fork. Transfer to a plate and cover to keep warm.

3. In the same skillet, heat the remaining 1 teaspoon of olive oil, swirling the bottom to coat. Add the spinach, ginger, and garlic, and cook, stirring constantly, for 2 minutes, or until the spinach begins to wilt. Remove the skillet from the heat.

4. Add the balsamic vinegar and lime juice to the spinach and stir. Divide the spinach among four plates and top each serving with a halibut fillet. Serve immediately.

INGREDIENT TIP To save time, you can purchase minced ginger and minced garlic in the produce section of most grocery stores. Simply store them in the refrigerator once opened.

Nutrition (per serving) Calories: 162; Total Fat: 6g; Saturated Fat: 1g; Cholesterol: 35mg; Sodium: 84mg; Potassium: 672mg; Magnesium: 120mg; Total Carbohydrates: 3g; Fiber: 1g; Sugars: 0g; Protein: 24g

Baked Flounder Packets with Summer Squash

SERVES 4 • PREP TIME: 5 MINUTES • COOK TIME: 10 MINUTES

This no-fuss dish is low in calories, yet packed with nutrition and flavor. Summer squash like zucchini and yellow squash are available year-round and are very good sources of magnesium, folate, calcium, and potassium for a healthy blood pressure. This recipe is easy to scale up or down and works the same whether you are cooking for 1 or 14.

4 (6-ounce) flounder fillets, or other white fish

Freshly ground black pepper

2 medium zucchini, sliced into thin rounds

2 medium yellow summer squash, sliced into thin rounds

1 medium red onion, sliced

2 tablespoons olive oil

2 tablespoons freshly squeezed lemon juice

1 lemon, thinly sliced

2 teaspoons dried basil

1. Preheat the oven to 450°F. Prepare four 12-by-18-inch sheets of aluminum foil. Spray the center of each sheet of foil with nonstick cooking spray.

2. Season the fish with the black pepper. Place one fish fillet on each piece of foil.

3. Arrange the zucchini, squash, and onion slices around each fillet. Drizzle ½ tablespoon of olive oil and ½ tablespoon of lemon juice onto the vegetables and fish.

4. Arrange a few lemon slices on top of each fillet and top each piece with ½ teaspoon of dried basil.

5. Bring up the sides of the foil and fold the tops over twice. Seal the ends, leaving room for air to circulate inside the packet. Set the packets on a rimmed baking sheet, and bake for 8 minutes. Carefully open one packet to check the fish and test with a fork to see if it flakes easily.

6. Serve immediately, using caution when opening the packets as the steam will be very hot.

SUBSTITUTION TIP Just about any type of fresh or dried herb works well with fish. Some good options for white fish include parsley, ginger, cumin, coriander, and cayenne.

Nutrition (per serving) Calories: 233; Total Fat: 9g; Saturated Fat: 1g; Cholesterol: 98mg; Sodium: 130mg; Potassium: 273mg; Magnesium: 24mg; Total Carbohydrates: 10g; Fiber: 4g; Sugars: 3g; Protein: 32g

Pecan-Crusted Catfish

SERVES 4 • PREP TIME: 5 MINUTES • COOK TIME: 20 MINUTES

Catfish is a good source of high-quality protein as well as beneficial omega-3 fatty acids that reduce inflammation in the body. Pecans are rich in cholesterol-lowering fiber and the minerals calcium, magnesium, and potassium, plus the nuts give the fish a crunchy, tasty coating. Serve this simple dish with a fresh salad of mixed greens and vegetables.

4 catfish fillets (approximately 1 pound)

½ teaspoon freshly ground black pepper

½ teaspoon garlic powder

2 teaspoons dried rosemary

2 egg whites, beaten

¾ cup pecans, chopped

Lemon wedges for serving

1. Preheat the oven to 400°F.

2. Line a baking sheet with foil and coat the foil with nonstick cooking spray.

3. Sprinkle the catfish fillets with the black pepper, garlic, and rosemary, then dip each fillet into the egg whites to coat.

4. Place the chopped pecans on a plate and press the egg-coated fillets firmly into the pecans, turning to coat both sides. Place the fillets on the baking sheet.

5. Bake for 20 minutes or until the fish flakes easily with a fork.

6. Serve with lemon wedges and enjoy.

INGREDIENT TIP The majority of the proteins in eggs are found in the whites, which are what coagulate and holds the coating on when cooked. You can also substitute milk in place of egg whites.

Nutrition (per serving) Calories: 263; Total Fat: 20g; Saturated Fat: 2g; Cholesterol: 47mg; Sodium: 228mg; Potassium: 104mg; Magnesium: 28mg; Total Carbohydrates: 4g; Fiber: 3g; Sugars: 1g; Protein: 18g

Chicken Legs with Rice and Peas

SERVES 4 • PREP TIME: 5 MINUTES • COOK TIME: 45 MINUTES

This delicious and easy recipe for chicken legs uses a flavorful seasoning mix of garlic and paprika as a coating for the chicken. Delectably baked, crispy, juicy, and tender, the sauce imparts a smoky flavor that is complemented by a side of rice and peas. This dish is full of B vitamins and protein. Just be sure to remove the skin before eating to keep unhealthy fats in check.

4 chicken drumsticks

3 tablespoons olive oil

4 garlic cloves, chopped

1 tablespoon paprika

1 teaspoon
dried oregano

1 cup instant
brown rice

2 ¾ cup frozen peas

1. Preheat the oven to 425°F.

2. Place the drumsticks in a 9-by-13-inch baking dish.

3. In a small skillet, heat the olive oil over medium heat. Add the garlic, paprika, and oregano. Cook for 1 minute, and remove from the heat.

4. Pour the mixture over the drumsticks and turn to coat evenly. Bake for about 45 minutes, or until an instant-read thermometer reads 180°F.

5. While the chicken bakes, cook the rice according to the package directions. When the rice has 7 minutes of cook time remaining, stir in the peas and re-cover.

6. Divide the rice among four plates and top each with a drumstick, skin removed.

Nutrition (per serving) Calories: 345; Total Fat: 15g; Saturated Fat: 2g; Cholesterol: 48mg; Sodium: 96mg; Potassium: 279mg; Magnesium: 88mg; Total Carbohydrates: 40g; Fiber: 4g; Sugars: 2g; Protein: 18g

Coconut Chicken Curry

SERVES 4 • PREP TIME: 10 MINUTES • COOK TIME: 45 MINUTES

Indian-inspired dishes are often very high in fat and calories because of the use of oil as well as regular coconut milk. By being careful with these two ingredients and using light coconut milk and less oil, you can cut hundreds of calories and reduce the amount of harmful fats while still maintaining flavor. Full of ingredients packed with fiber, vitamins, and minerals, this delicious dish brings together all of the classic flavors of traditional Indian cuisine to the DASH diet.

1 cup brown jasmine rice

2 cups water

2 teaspoons olive oil

2 garlic cloves, minced

2 tablespoons minced fresh ginger

1 tablespoon curry powder

1 medium apple, peel on, cored and diced

1 tablespoon honey

½ cup low-fat/light coconut milk

¾ cup low-sodium chicken broth

1 pound boneless, skinless chicken breast, cut into bite-size cubes

¼ cup chopped unsalted cashews

2 tablespoons golden raisins

4 tablespoons chopped fresh cilantro leaves

1. In a medium saucepan with a tight-fitting lid, combine the rice and water, and bring to a boil. Stir once, cover, and reduce heat to low. Simmer for 30 to 35 minutes. Do not lift the lid or stir.

2. Meanwhile, heat the olive oil in a large skillet over medium heat. Add the garlic and sauté for 1 minute. Add the ginger and curry powder and mix well, cooking for 1 minute.

3. Add the apple, honey, coconut milk, and broth, reduce the heat to medium, and cook for about 3 minutes.

4. Add the chicken to the pan, stir all the ingredients, and cover the pan. Simmer over medium-low heat until the chicken is cooked through and an instant-read thermometer registers 165°F, about 30 minutes.

5. Add the cashews and raisins and stir in the cilantro.

6. Fluff the rice with a fork. Serve the chicken over the rice.

INGREDIENT TIP Ginger root must be peeled before using. Unpeeled ginger root will only keep for about one week in the refrigerator. You can tell it's no longer fresh when the skin begins to wrinkle. It also doesn't freeze well, so it's best to buy just the amount you need for a particular recipe.

Nutrition (per serving) Calories: 439; Total Fat 12g; Saturated Fat: 4g; Cholesterol: 65mg; Sodium: 69mg; Potassium: 114mg; Magnesium: 8mg; Total Carbohydrates: 51g; Fiber: 4g; Sugars: 11g; Protein: 31g

Fajita-Style
Beef Tacos,
page 120

Beef & Pork Entrées

Simple Herb-Roasted Pork Loin and Potatoes

SERVES 4 • PREP TIME: 5 MINUTES • COOK TIME: 1 HOUR

This simple recipe for pork loin is perfect for baking on a Sunday afternoon, so you have a nutritious dinner as well as leftovers for busy weekday lunches. Not to be confused with pork tenderloin, pork loin is a larger cut of meat, so you can get it to order. A lean, mild-flavored meat, pork loin is best slow-roasted in the oven. Take advantage of the oven time to roast your favorite vegetables as a nutritious side.

1 (1-pound) pork loin, trimmed

8 garlic cloves

¼ cup olive oil, divided

Freshly ground black pepper

1 cup cubed raw sweet potato

1 cup small gold potatoes, quartered

8 fresh thyme sprigs, chopped

1. Preheat the oven to 350°F. Rub the pork with the garlic and 2 tablespoons of the olive oil. Season with the black pepper. Coat a 9-by-13-inch baking dish with nonstick cooking spray.

2. Place the pork in the prepared baking dish. Bake for approximately 60 minutes, or until an instant-read thermometer inserted in the center registers 145°F.

3. Twenty minutes into the cooking time, place the cubed and sliced sweet potatoes and gold potatoes on a rimmed baking dish, drizzle with the remaining olive oil, sprinkle with the thyme, and place in the oven. The potatoes should be finished roasting about the same time as the pork and should be tender and slightly browned.

4. Once the pork is finished cooking, remove from the oven and let the meat stand for 15 minutes before carving. Cut into eight slices. Serve with the roasted potatoes and a green salad.

INGREDIENT TIP Pork loin goes by a few other names, including center-cut pork-loin roast, center-cut pork roast, pork-center loin roast, pork-center-cut rib roast, pork-loin center cut, and pork-loin rib half. It can be sold bone-in or boneless.

Nutrition (per serving) Total Calories: 426; Total Fat: 22g; Saturated Fat: 5g; Cholesterol: 45mg; Sodium: 56mg; Potassium: 858mg; Magnesium: 48mg; Total Carbohydrates: 21g; Fiber: 4g; Sugars: 3g; Protein: 27g

Tuscan Pork Kebabs

SERVES 4 • PREP TIME: 15 MINUTES • COOK TIME: 10 MINUTES

The DASH diet recommends decreasing your consumption of red meat and treating it as more of a side dish or treat than the main feature of the meal. It's easy to do this when you focus on filling your plate with vegetables, and with this recipe for pork kebabs, you can load up your skewers with your favorite veggies, while keeping the meat portion in check.

4 teaspoons olive oil, plus 1 tablespoon

1 tablespoon lemon zest

½ teaspoon freshly ground black pepper

2 garlic cloves, crushed

1 pound pork tenderloin, trimmed and cut into 1-inch pieces

16 (1-inch) pieces red bell pepper

16 button mushrooms

8 cups chopped, stemmed spinach

1. Prepare the grill to medium-high heat, or preheat the broiler to high, for at least 5 minutes.

2. Combine 4 teaspoons of the olive oil, lemon zest, black pepper, and garlic in a large bowl, stirring well. Add the pork, and marinate at room temperature for 15 minutes, tossing occasionally.

3. Thread the pork, bell peppers, and mushrooms alternately onto each of the eight 8-inch skewers. Place the skewers on a grill rack coated with cooking spray, and grill, turning occasionally, for 10 minutes, or until the pork is no longer pink and is completely cooked. If using the broiler, place the skewers under the broiler and cook for 5 minutes, or until the edges begin to brown, then rotate and cook for an additional 5 minutes.

4. While the pork cooks, heat a large skillet over medium-high heat. Add 1 tablespoon of the olive oil to the pan, and swirl to coat. Add the spinach and sauté for 5 minutes until the spinach wilts.

5. Serve the spinach alongside the kebabs.

SUBSTITUTION TIP Another way to enjoy red meat as a "treat" while utilizing this recipe is to use less pork and alternate the pieces of pork on the skewers with pieces of chicken breast or shrimp.

Nutrition (per serving) Calories: 251; Total Fat: 14g; Saturated Fat: 3g; Cholesterol: 45mg; Sodium: 88mg; Potassium: 682mg; Magnesium: 60mg; Total Carbohydrates: 11g; Fiber: 3g; Sugars: 4g; Protein: 24g

Pork and Vegetable Stew

SERVES 4 • PREP TIME: 10 MINUTES • COOK TIME: 35 MINUTES

This Ukrainian-style one-pot stew is as vibrant as it is delicious and nutritious. You can throw it together in just over 30 minutes, which makes it perfect for busy weeknights. It packs a big nutritional punch with potassium-rich potatoes, nutrient-filled carrots, and protein-rich meat.

2 tablespoons olive oil

1 medium onion, chopped

1 pound pork tenderloin, cut into thin strips

4 carrots, thinly sliced

2 teaspoons dried thyme

4 garlic cloves, minced

2 red potatoes, cubed

½ cup low-sodium chicken stock

1. Heat the olive oil in a large nonstick skillet over medium heat. Add the onion and cook for 5 to 7 minutes, or until the onions are translucent.

2. Add the pork and continue cooking for 10 minutes. Add the carrots, thyme, and garlic, and cook for another 5 minutes.

3. Add the potatoes and chicken stock and cover with a lid. Bring to a boil and simmer for 10 to 15 minutes, stirring occasionally until the potatoes are cooked through, the flavors have blended, and the pork is cooked through and no longer pink. Pork tenderloin should be cooked to an internal temperature of 145°F to160°F.

4. Serve immediately.

SUBSTITUTION TIP If you'd like your stew to be a little thinner, add 1 to 2 (14-ounce) cans of no-salt diced tomatoes to the pot when you add the potatoes.

Nutrition (per serving) Calories: 289; Total Fat: 12g; Saturated Fat: 3g; Cholesterol: 45mg; Sodium: 89mg; Potassium: 566mg; Magnesium: 12mg; Total Carbohydrates: 24g; Fiber: 4g; Sugars: 3g; Protein: 22g

Pork and Cabbage Stir-Fry

SERVES 4 • PREP TIME: 5 MINUTES • COOK TIME: 10 MINUTES

Stir-fry recipes are quick-and-easy dinners that can use up any meat or vegetable leftovers in the refrigerator. This recipe uses boneless pork chops, frozen snap peas, and ground ginger and garlic for seasoning in place of high-sodium soy sauce. Full of fiber and heart-healthy B vitamins, snap peas boost the magnesium and potassium content of this nutritious dish.

1 pound boneless pork chops, cut into ½-inch thick pieces and trimmed of visible fat

1 teaspoon ground ginger

1 teaspoon garlic powder

1 (16-ounce) package frozen snap peas (or stir-fry vegetables), thawed

2 cups shredded purple cabbage

2 cups cooked brown rice, warm

1. Coat a skillet with nonstick cooking spray and heat over high heat. Add the pork, ginger, and garlic, and stir-fry for 1 minute.

2. Add the snap peas, stirring constantly, for 2 to 3 minutes, or until the pork is fully cooked and the snap peas are warmed. Remove the skillet from the heat, and transfer the pork and snap peas to a medium bowl.

3. Spray the skillet with nonstick cooking spray again. Heat over high heat and add the shredded cabbage. Stir-fry for 3 to 4 minutes, or until the cabbage is wilted.

continued >

4. Remove the skillet from the heat, and return the pork and snap peas to the skillet. Stir to combine.

5. Divide the rice among four plates and top with equal portions of the pork and cabbage. Serve immediately.

SUBSTITUTION TIP For an even more DASH-friendly, veggie-rich dish, serve over cooked riced cauliflower instead of brown rice. Riced cauliflower can be found in the produce and freezer sections at your grocery store. This substitution will also significantly lower the calorie count.

Nutrition (per serving) Calories: 287; Total Fat: 7g; Saturated Fat: 3g; Cholesterol: 45mg; Sodium: 273mg; Potassium: 279mg; Magnesium: 52mg; Total Carbohydrates: 30g; Fiber: 5g; Sugars: 3g; Protein: 25g

Pork and Black Bean Quesadillas

SERVES 4 • PREP TIME: 5 MINUTES • COOK TIME: 25 MINUTES

This recipe helps you meet your DASH-recommended daily servings of beans. Black beans are full of fiber, plant protein, and blood pressure–lowering minerals calcium and magnesium. Corn tortillas are used in place of wheat to keep the sodium levels in check. With added calcium from low-fat cheese, the quesadillas are great with sliced avocado or your favorite toppings.

2 tablespoons olive oil

1 cup diced pork tenderloin

1 cup sliced mushrooms

1 teaspoon ground cumin

1 teaspoon ground oregano

1 (15-ounce) can black beans, drained and rinsed

16 corn tortillas

2 cups grated low-fat Mexican cheese blend

¼ cup chopped fresh cilantro

4 tomato or avocado slices (optional)

1. Heat the olive oil in a large skillet over medium heat. Add the pork and cook for 5 minutes.

2. Add the mushrooms, cumin, and oregano, and cook for another 10 minutes.

3. Add the beans and continue cooking for another 5 to 10 minutes, or until the pork is cooked through and no longer pink, and then remove the skillet from the heat. Pork tenderloin should be cooked to an internal temperature of 145°F to 160°F.

4. On a large plate or tray, place eight tortillas. Divide the bean-and-pork mixture evenly between the eight tortillas, sprinkle with 1 cup of the cheese, and place another tortilla on top.

continued >

Pork and Black Bean Quesadillas *continued*

5. Wipe out the skillet with a paper towel and heat over medium-high heat. Carefully place one quesadilla in the skillet and cook on one side until nicely browned, about 2 to 3 minutes. Turn and brown the other side for 2 to 3 minutes. Remove to a cutting board and cut into four wedges. Repeat with the remaining quesadillas.

6. Serve with fresh cilantro, and avocado or tomato slices (if using).

SUBSTITUTION TIP You can use whole-wheat tortillas in place of the corn if you prefer a more traditional quesadilla. Just keep in mind that whole-wheat tortillas are higher in sodium than corn tortillas, so just balance this choice out with your other choices throughout the day.

Nutrition (per serving) Calories: 527; Total Fat: 25g; Saturated Fat: 2g; Cholesterol: 33mg; Sodium: 592mg; Potassium: 61mg; Magnesium: 38mg; Total Carbohydrates: 42g; Fiber: 7g; Sugars: 0g; Protein: 36g

Pork with Vegetables and Pasta

SERVES 4 • PREP TIME: 10 MINUTES • COOK TIME: 25 MINUTES

This terrific combination of nutritious ingredients helps you meet a number of your daily DASH-recommended food-group servings. Whole-wheat ziti is full of fiber, asparagus provides potassium, cheese boosts the calcium content, and lean pork provides high-quality protein.

5 ounces
whole-wheat ziti

2 tablespoons plus
1 teaspoon olive oil

1 large red bell
pepper, chopped

2 cups chopped
asparagus

3 garlic cloves, minced

1 teaspoon
dried oregano

8 ounces pork
tenderloin,
cut into strips

1 (15-ounce) can
no-salt crushed
tomatoes

½ teaspoon freshly
ground black pepper

½ cup shredded low-fat
mozzarella cheese

1. Preheat the oven to 375°F.

2. Cook the ziti according to the package directions. Drain and return the pasta to the pot. Add 1 teaspoon of the olive oil and toss to coat.

3. Heat the remaining 2 tablespoons of olive oil in a large skillet over medium heat. Add the bell pepper, asparagus, garlic, and oregano. Cook for 4 to 5 minutes until the vegetables are soft.

4. Stir in the pork and cook until the pork is browned, 2 to 3 minutes per side. Stir in the tomatoes and cook for 2 minutes. Season with the black pepper.

5. Add the pasta to the skillet and toss to combine. Pour into a shallow 2.5- or 3-quart baking dish. Sprinkle with the cheese. Bake until heated through and the cheese is melted and slightly browned, about 20 minutes.

INGREDIENT TIP To reduce the sodium content further, use 2 cups of fresh chopped tomatoes in place of 1 (15-ounce) can.

Nutrition (per serving) Calories: 299; Total Fat: 8g; Saturated Fat: 2g; Cholesterol: 25mg; Sodium: 173mg; Potassium: 524mg; Magnesium: 32mg; Total Carbohydrates: 37g; Fiber: 6g; Sugars: 2g; Protein: 21g

Pork Medallions with Herbs

SERVES 2 • PREP TIME: 5 MINUTES • COOK TIME: 10 MINUTES

This quick and delicious recipe for pork medallions uses a flavorful mix of dried herbs called herbes de Provence, which includes thyme, marjoram, rosemary, basil, fennel, sage, and lavender. Paired with a quick sauté of potassium-rich and magnesium-rich spinach with walnuts, this recipe makes a speedy DASH dinner.

8 ounces pork tenderloin, trimmed of visible fat and cut crosswise into 6 pieces

Freshly ground black pepper

2 teaspoons olive oil

4 cups baby spinach

1 teaspoon herbes de Provence

¼ cup dry white wine

2 tablespoons chopped walnuts

1. Season the pork with the black pepper. Place the pork between two sheets of waxed paper and pound the meat with a mallet or roll it with a rolling pin until it is about ¼ inch thick.

2. In a large nonstick frying pan, add the olive oil and cook the pork over medium-high heat until browned on one side, 2 to 3 minutes. Turn the meat, add the spinach, and cook for an additional 2 to 3 minutes until the meat is browned on the second side and the spinach is wilted. Remove from the heat and season with herbes de Provence. Place the pork and spinach on individual plates and keep warm.

3. Pour the wine into the frying pan, and bring to a boil. Scrape the brown bits from the bottom of the pan. Pour the wine sauce over the pork, top with the chopped walnuts, and serve immediately.

SUBSTITUTION TIP If you don't have herbes de Provence, simply substitute with 1 teaspoon of your favorite dried herbs or use a combination of the herbs mentioned in the head note.

Nutrition (per serving) Calories: 273; Total Fat: 15g; Saturated Fat: 3g; Cholesterol: 45mg; Sodium: 87mg; Potassium: 415mg; Magnesium: 64mg; Total Carbohydrates: 5g; Fiber: 2g; Sugars: 0g; Protein: 22g

Beef Tenderloin with Balsamic Tomatoes

SERVES 2 • PREP TIME: 5 MINUTES • COOK TIME: 20 MINUTES

Beef tenderloin is an excellent source of high-quality protein, heart-healthy B vitamins, and important minerals including zinc, iron, magnesium, and potassium. Keep an eye on beef portion sizes and serve with a large fresh spinach salad and a side of steamed vegetables for a speedy, delicious, and nutritious meal.

½ cup balsamic vinegar

¾ cup coarsely chopped, seeded tomato

2 teaspoons olive oil

2 (3- to 4-ounce, ¾-inch-thick) beef tenderloin steaks, trimmed of visible fat

1 teaspoon fresh thyme (or ½ teaspoon dried)

1. In a small saucepan, bring the balsamic vinegar to a boil. Reduce the heat and simmer, uncovered, for 5 minutes, or until the liquid is reduced to ¼ cup. Stir in the tomatoes and cook for 1 to 2 minutes more. Remove the saucepan from the heat.

2. In a large skillet, heat the olive oil over medium-high heat. Add the steaks, and reduce the heat to medium. Cook the steaks to desired doneness, turning once. Allow 7 to 9 minutes per side for medium (160°F).

3. Spoon the balsamic tomatoes over the steaks, and sprinkle with the thyme. Serve immediately.

INGREDIENT TIP Balsamic vinegar's tangy and sweet properties make it an adaptable, low-sodium ingredient to keep on hand for your DASH diet. Very low in calories and sodium, and with with no fat, balsamic vinegar is rich in phytonutrients and contains numerous minerals, including calcium, magnesium, and potassium.

Nutrition (per serving) Calories: 298; Total Fat: 20g; Saturated Fat: 7g; Cholesterol: 58mg; Sodium: 69mg; Potassium: 407mg; Magnesium: 24mg; Total Carbohydrates: 11g; Fiber: 1g; Sugars: 0g; Protein: 17g

Fajita-Style Beef Tacos

SERVES 4 • PREP TIME: 5 MINUTES • COOK TIME: 15 MINUTES

Intensely flavorful and spicy, but not too hot, these steak fajitas are ready fast. Bell peppers are the perfect vegetable for stir-frying, as they keep their firm consistency when heated and provide a flavor that is a bit sweet while still being savory. Combined with flavorful red onion, this healthy high-protein and nutrient-rich dish makes a speedy supper.

1 tablespoon olive oil

1 red bell pepper, sliced and deseeded

1 medium red onion, sliced

12 ounces flank steak, trimmed of fat, sliced into thin strips

½ teaspoon chili powder

1 teaspoon cumin

8 (6-inch) whole-wheat flour tortillas, warmed

1 avocado, peeled, seeded, and cubed

¼ cup fresh cilantro

¼ cup feta cheese

4 lime wedges (optional)

1. Heat the olive oil in a large skillet over medium-high heat, about 2 minutes. Add the bell peppers and onion and cook, stirring often, until just tender, about 5 minutes. Remove the vegetables from the skillet.

2. Add the steak slices to the same skillet. Stir-fry for 2 to 3 minutes, or until no longer raw.

3. Return the vegetables to the skillet, add the chili powder and cumin, and stir-fry for 2 to 3 minutes, or until heated through.

4. Spoon the fajita filling into warm tortillas, and top with equal portions of avocado, cilantro, and a sprinkle of feta.

5. Serve immediately with fresh limes (if using).

SUBSTITUTION TIP You can lower the sodium content and calories in this recipe while boosting the fiber, vitamins, and minerals by serving the fajitas in romaine lettuce leaves, or over mixed baby greens, instead of using the tortillas.

Nutrition (per serving) Calories: 456; Total Fat: 23g; Saturated Fat: 6g; Cholesterol: 35mg; Sodium: 745mg; Potassium: 560mg; Magnesium: 36mg; Total Carbohydrates: 37g; Fiber: 21g; Sugars: 3g; Protein: 36g

Steak Dijon with Green Beans

SERVES 4 • PREP TIME: 5 MINUTES • COOK TIME: 20 MINUTES

This delicious recipe gives steak Dijon a healthy boost by pairing it with nutrient-rich green beans, and infusing the dish with bold flavor by topping it with a quick-to-prepare mustard sauce. Serve it over mixed baby greens for added blood pressure–lowering minerals, and consider a side of a baked sweet potato for an all-around meal.

1 tablespoon olive oil

12 ounces flank steak, trimmed of fat

½ teaspoon freshly ground black pepper, divided

1 medium onion, sliced

1 cup no-salt chicken broth

2 tablespoons finely chopped fresh dill

1 tablespoon Dijon mustard

1 pound microwave-in-bag green beans

8 cups mixed baby greens or baby spinach

1. In a large skillet, heat the olive oil over medium-high heat. Season the steaks with ¼ teaspoon of the black pepper, and add the steak to the skillet. Cook until desired doneness: 5 to 7 minutes per side for medium (140°F), or 8 to 10 minutes for medium-well (150°F). Transfer the steak to a cutting board. Cover loosely with foil.

2. In the same skillet, cook the onion for 2 minutes, stirring constantly. Stir in the broth, and heat to simmering. Allow to simmer for 5 minutes, and then whisk in the dill, mustard, and remaining pepper. Transfer to a small bowl.

3. Prepare the green beans according to the package directions.

4. Slice the steak and serve alongside the green beans and baby greens in four equal portions. Serve the sauce on the side.

Nutrition (per serving) Calories: 226; Total Fat: 10g; Saturated Fat: 3g; Cholesterol: 30mg; Sodium: 201mg; Potassium: 896mg; Magnesium: 100mg; Total Carbohydrates: 13g; Fiber: 6g; Sugars: 0g; Protein: 22g

Balsamic Grilled Steak Salad with Peaches

SERVES 4 • PREP TIME: 15 MINUTES • COOK TIME: 15 MINUTES

One strategy for increasing your daily servings of vegetables is to include more meal-size salads in your menu. Eating more salads and vegetables, and keeping meat-based meals in check, is a proven weight-loss strategy, and it is made easy by this nutritious and delicious recipe. Peaches provide additional vitamins, minerals, and fiber, and add a contrast to the savory grilled steak.

12 ounces flank steak, trimmed of fat

¼ cup balsamic vinegar

2 garlic cloves, minced

1 tablespoon brown sugar

3 tablespoons olive oil, divided

Freshly ground black pepper

Juice of 1 lemon

8 cups fresh baby spinach

2 peaches, pitted and thinly sliced

1 English cucumber, sliced

1. Place the steak in a large resealable plastic bag or baking dish and add the balsamic vinegar, garlic, and sugar. Allow to marinate for 15 minutes.

2. Heat a grill or grill pan to high. Remove the steak from the marinade, and rub it with 1 tablespoon of the olive oil and season with the black pepper.

3. Grill the steak until desired doneness: 5 to 7 minutes per side for medium (140°F), or 8 to 10 minutes for medium-well (150°F). Let the steak rest for 5 minutes before slicing.

4. Meanwhile, in a small bowl, whisk together the remaining 2 tablespoons of olive oil and the lemon juice, and season to taste with the black pepper.

5. In a large bowl, toss together the spinach, peaches, cucumber, and steak. Drizzle with the lemon-oil dressing, and gently toss.

6. Serve immediately.

SUBSTITUTION TIP A peppery green like arugula would work well in this recipe, too; the spicy flavor would make a great contrast to the sweet peaches. Like all dark leafy greens, arugula is high in calcium, magnesium, and potassium. This green is also known as rocket salad, roquette, and rucola.

Nutrition (per serving) Calories: 287; Total Fat: 17g; Saturated Fat: 4g; Cholesterol: 30mg; Sodium: 100mg; Potassium: 724mg; Magnesium: 72mg; Total Carbohydrates: 15g; Fiber: 3g; Sugars: 9g; Protein: 21g

Steak and Potatoes

SERVES 2 • PREP TIME: 5 MINUTES • COOK TIME: 20 MINUTES

This classic combination uses the flavors of dill to season sirloin steaks, which are trimmed to keep unhealthy fats in check. Russet potatoes are swapped in favor of small red potatoes, whose skin contains two to three times the antioxidant power of white potatoes. Because you don't peel red potatoes, you also get more fiber. Potatoes are one of the best sources of blood pressure–lowering potassium. Serve this dish with a side of green vegetables.

½ pound small red potatoes (about 8)

2 tablespoons olive oil, divided

2 small skirt steaks (such as sirloin or top round, about 8 ounces total)

Freshly ground black pepper

2 scallions, sliced

¼ cup fresh chopped dill

2 tablespoons white wine vinegar

1. Place the potatoes in a large pot. Add enough cold water to cover and bring to a boil. Reduce the heat and simmer for 15 to 18 minutes, or until just tender. Drain the potatoes and run them under cold water to cool. Cut the potatoes in half. Set aside.

2. While the potatoes are cooking, heat 1 tablespoon of the olive oil in a large skillet over medium-high heat. Season the steaks with the black pepper, and add the steak to the skillet. Cook until desired doneness: 5 to 7 minutes per side for medium (140°F), or 8 to 10 minutes for medium-well (150°F).

3. In a large bowl, combine the scallions, dill, white wine vinegar, and remaining 1 tablespoon of the olive oil. Add the potatoes and toss to coat.

4. Divide the steak and potatoes among two plates, and serve immediately.

INGREDIENT TIP For even more Mediterranean flavor, fold 1 ounce of feta cheese in with the potatoes. Feta cheese is fairly high in sodium, so if you do add it, keep in mind that the sodium content of this dish will be higher. Just balance it out with your other choices throughout the day.

Nutrition (per serving) Calories: 440; Total Fat: 26g; Saturated Fat: 7g; Cholesterol: 67mg; Sodium: 107mg; Potassium: 842mg; Magnesium: 28mg; Total Carbohydrates: 19g; Fiber: 3g; Sugars: 2g; Protein: 33g

Steak with Chickpeas and Spinach

SERVES 4 • PREP TIME: 5 MINUTES • COOK TIME: 15 MINUTES

This DASH-friendly dish includes beans, greens, and lean protein in a quick-to-prepare recipe full of flavor. The DASH diet recommends four to five servings of beans and legumes each week to reap their heart-healthy benefits—and this dish will help you on your way. It is full of cholesterol-lowering fiber, B vitamins, minerals, and protein.

1 teaspoon olive oil, plus 2 tablespoons

12 ounces flank steak

Freshly ground black pepper

1 (15-ounce) can chickpeas, drained and rinsed

¼ cup fresh mint

2 scallions, sliced

1 tablespoon freshly squeezed lemon juice

8 cups baby spinach

1. Heat 1 teaspoon of the olive oil in a large skillet over medium-high heat.

2. Season the steak with black pepper, and add the steak to the skillet. Cook to the desired doneness: 5 to 7 minutes per side for medium (140°F), or 8 to 10 minutes for medium-well (150°F). Let the steak rest for 5 minutes before slicing.

3. Meanwhile, in a large bowl, combine the chickpeas, mint, scallions, lemon juice, and the remaining 2 tablespoons of olive oil. Fold in the spinach. Season with the black pepper.

4. Slice the steak and divide among four plates. Serve an equal portion of the salad alongside the steak.

SUBSTITUTION TIP You can use any type of bean in this recipe. When using canned beans, whether or not salt has been added, always drain the beans in a colander and rinse under cold water to remove as much of the sodium as possible. (Yes, there is some salt in canned beans labeled "no-salt.")

Nutrition (per serving) Calories: 319; Total Fat: 15g; Saturated Fat: 4g; Cholesterol: 30mg; Sodium: 201mg; Potassium: 634mg; Magnesium: 49mg; Total Carbohydrates: 19g; Fiber: 8g; Sugars: 0g; Protein: 26g

Southwestern Meatballs

SERVES 4 • PREP TIME: 5 MINUTES • COOK TIME: 20 MINUTES

These meatballs are full of Southwestern flavor from finely chopped corn tortillas, smoky chipotle chili, onion, and garlic. Made using lean ground sirloin, these delicious meatballs pair well with a side of rice, sautéed squash, and avocado slices.

2 tablespoons olive oil, divided

½ cup diced onion

2 garlic cloves, minced

½ cup finely chopped corn tortillas (about 2 to 3 tortillas)

1 tablespoon minced chipotle chilies in adobe sauce

½ teaspoon oregano

½ teaspoon freshly ground black pepper

½ cup chopped fresh cilantro

1 large egg

12 ounces 93% lean ground round

1. Heat a nonstick skillet over medium heat. Add 1 tablespoon of the olive oil to the skillet. Add the onion and minced garlic, and cook for 4 minutes. Stir in the chopped corn tortillas, chipotle chilies, oregano, and black pepper. Cook for 3 minutes.

2. Transfer the mixture to a medium bowl. Stir in the cilantro and egg. Add the ground meat, and mix well to combine.

3. Using your hands, form the mixture into 12 balls.

4. Return the skillet to the heat, and add the remaining oil. Place the meatballs in the skillet, and cook for 6 minutes. Cover and cook for 4 more minutes.

5. Serve immediately.

BUDGET-SAVER TIP Ground round is generally the leanest ground beef. Check the label and choose a variety that is 90% lean or 93% lean, which means that the meat contains only 10% and 7% fat, respectively.

Nutrition (per serving) Calories: 264; Total Fat: 14g; Saturated Fat: 4g; Cholesterol: 95mg; Sodium: 123mg; Potassium: 61mg; Magnesium: 32mg; Total Carbohydrates: 10g; Fiber: 1g; Sugars: 0g; Protein: 21g

Banana–Chocolate
Chip Muffins,
page 144

CHAPTER
8

Snacks, Sides & Desserts

Peach Hummus

YIELD: 2 CUPS • PREP TIME: 10 MINUTES

Homemade hummus is very easy to make and is a nutritious and filling snack you can enjoy on your DASH eating plan. Made using canned chickpeas (garbanzo beans), sesame paste, and seasonings, you can blend in a variety of fruits and vegetables to create endless variations. This recipe incorporates canned peaches to create a mildly sweet and zesty dip.

1 (15-ounce) can chickpeas (garbanzo beans), drained and rinsed

¼ cup tahini

1 (15-ounce) can peaches in light juice, drained, divided

2 tablespoons olive oil

2 to 3 tablespoons water

1 small clove garlic, minced

¼ cup freshly squeezed lemon juice (1 large lemon)

½ teaspoon ground cumin

2 tablespoons chopped fresh cilantro, for garnish (optional)

1. In a blender or food processor, combine the chickpeas, tahini, half of the peaches, olive oil, water, garlic, lemon juice, and cumin. Blend until smooth. Transfer the mixture to a serving bowl.

2. Chop the remaining peaches into chunks.

3. Top the hummus with the peach chunks and cilantro (if using) before serving.

SUBSTITUTION TIP If you don't have tahini (a paste made from sesame seeds), you can leave it out and your hummus will still be delicious. Just add 1 to 2 tablespoons of additional olive oil. Another option is to use ¼ cup of a natural unsweetened creamy peanut butter in its place.

Nutrition (¼ cup) Calories: 153; Total Fat: 8g; Saturated Fat: 1g; Cholesterol: 0mg; Sodium: 65mg; Potassium: 97mg; Magnesium: 35mg; Total Carbohydrates: 18g; Fiber: 4g; Sugars: 0g; Protein: 5g

Roasted Edamame

SERVES 6 • PREP TIME: 5 MINUTES • COOK TIME: 25 MINUTES

Utterly addictive and delicious, roasted edamame (green soybeans) is one snack you can enjoy guilt-free. They are low in fat and calories and are loaded with the perfect energy-boosting mix of carbohydrates, protein, and fiber. This quick-and-simple recipe turns a frozen food into a nutritious snack in minutes.

1 (12-ounce) bag frozen, shelled edamame

1 tablespoon olive oil

½ teaspoon freshly ground black pepper

½ teaspoon onion powder

½ teaspoon garlic powder

2 to 3 tablespoons Parmesan cheese (optional)

1. Preheat the oven to 425°F. Rinse the edamame in a strainer until any ice is melted and the beans are mostly thawed. Blot dry with paper towels.

2. In a medium bowl, whisk together the olive oil, black pepper, onion powder, garlic powder, and cheese (if using). Add the edamame and toss to combine.

3. Spread the edamame out on a baking sheet that has been lightly sprayed with cooking spray. Roast the edamame for 20 to 25 minutes (stirring halfway through) or until the beans are lightly browned and crispy.

4. Serve immediately.

INGREDIENT TIP Vary the seasonings to your likings. For spicy edamame, use ½ teaspoon of ground cayenne pepper and ½ teaspoon of garlic powder. You can also use 1 to 2 teaspoons of sriracha sauce for a real kick. For a sweet-and-spicy version, try 1 to 2 teaspoons of honey, ½ teaspoon of ground ginger, ½ teaspoon of garlic powder, and ½ teaspoon of ground cayenne.

Nutrition (per serving) Calories: 72; Total Fat: 4g; Saturated Fat: 0g; Cholesterol: 0mg; Sodium: 35mg; Potassium: 6mg; Magnesium: 8mg; Total Carbohydrates: 5g; Fiber: 1g; Sugars: 1g; Protein: 5g

Ricotta and Strawberry Bruschetta

SERVES 4 • PREP TIME: 15 MINUTES • COOK TIME: 8 MINUTES

*Bruschetta is an Italian appetizer of toasted garlic bread that is tradition-
ally topped with chopped tomatoes and olive oil. This recipe provides a
sweet-and-savory way to enjoy these bread-based bites while helping you
meet your DASH-recommended servings of whole grains, low-fat dairy,
and fruit. Small slices of toasted whole-grain bread are topped with lemony,
low-fat ricotta, and sprinkled with fresh strawberries accented with thyme.
Delicious and easy to make, enjoy this fruity take on bruschetta as a mid-
day snack.*

4 slices crusty
whole-grain bread

1 cup low-fat
ricotta cheese

½ teaspoon grated
lemon zest

½ cup sliced
strawberries

2 teaspoons
fresh thyme

1. Preheat the oven to 425°F. Place the bread slices
   on a large baking sheet. Bake until lightly toasted,
   about 8 minutes.

2. In a small bowl, stir together the ricotta and
   lemon zest.

3. Top each piece of toast with an equal amount of
   the ricotta mixture. Sprinkle the strawberry slices
   and thyme evenly over the top.

4. Serve immediately.

SUBSTITUTION TIP Substitute ½ cup of your favorite
berry in place of the strawberry slices. Or, for a more
traditional taste, chop ½ cup of tomatoes and mix with
1 to 2 garlic cloves (chopped), 2 teaspoons of olive oil,
and 1 tablespoon of chopped fresh basil.

Nutrition (per serving) Calories: 201; Total Fat: 5g;
Saturated Fat: 2g; Cholesterol: 15mg; Sodium: 340mg;
Potassium: 34mg; Magnesium: 24mg; Total Carbohydrates: 34g;
Fiber: 10g; Sugars: 9g; Protein: 11g

Avocado with Black Bean Salad

SERVES 4 • PREP TIME: 10 MINUTES

This quick-and-easy recipe is as appealing to the eye as it is satisfying and delicious. Creamy avocado is topped with seasoned black beans to create a side dish or snack rich in heart-healthy monounsaturated fats, plant-based protein, fiber, and blood pressure–lowering minerals. This recipe would even make a filling and balanced breakfast.

1 tablespoon freshly squeezed lime juice

1 tablespoon olive oil

1 (15-ounce) can black beans, drained and rinsed

½ green bell pepper, finely chopped

1 garlic clove, minced

¼ teaspoon freshly ground black pepper

2 teaspoons chopped fresh cilantro

1 avocado, peeled, pitted, and quartered

1. In a large bowl, add the lime juice and gradually whisk in the olive oil. Stir in the beans, bell pepper, garlic, black pepper, and cilantro.

2. Place the avocado, cut-sides up, on four serving plates. Spoon the bean mixture into the cavities so it overflows onto the plate.

3. Serve immediately.

SUBSTITUTION TIP You can replace the lime juice in this recipe with an equal amount of vinegar, or use a ½ tablespoon of each. Apple cider vinegar or white wine vinegar are good choices. Feel free to adjust the amount to taste.

Nutrition (per serving) Calories: 205; Total Fat: 11g; Saturated Fat: 1g; Cholesterol: 0mg; Sodium: 111mg; Potassium: 250mg; Magnesium: 36mg; Total Carbohydrates: 22g; Fiber: 9g; Sugars: 1g; Protein: 7g

Yogurt-Dill Smashed Potatoes

SERVES 4 • PREP TIME: 5 MINUTES • COOK TIME: 20 MINUTES

Potatoes are an excellent source of potassium and fiber. They also contain almost 30 mg of vitamin C. This smashed-potato recipe uses red potatoes, which have a thin skin that is left on for added antioxidants and plant nutrients. Low-fat yogurt keeps this dish healthy and high in calcium, with the creamy consistency you love.

1 pound small red potatoes, cleaned, unpeeled

½ cup diced red onion

1 cup plain low-fat yogurt

2 teaspoons dried dill

2 garlic cloves, minced

⅛ teaspoon freshly ground black pepper

1. Place the potatoes in a medium saucepan and add enough cold water to cover. Bring to a boil over medium-high heat.

2. Reduce the heat to simmer, and cook for 15 to 20 minutes, or until the potatoes are tender. Drain and allow to cool slightly.

3. Meanwhile, in a large bowl, combine the remaining ingredients, and mix well. Set aside.

4. Leaving the potato skins on, smash each potato using the bottom of a glass on a cutting board. Transfer the smashed potatoes to the yogurt dressing. When all of the potatoes have been smashed, stir to coat.

5. Serve immediately.

SUBSTITUTION TIP Small gold potatoes make a good substitution for red potatoes in this recipe. You might also consider using sweet potatoes. If you do use sweet potatoes, remove the skins.

Nutrition (per serving) Calories: 128; Total Fat: 1g; Saturated Fat: 1g; Cholesterol: 4mg; Sodium: 64mg; Potassium: 666mg; Magnesium: 36mg; Total Carbohydrates: 24g; Fiber: 3g; Sugars: 6g; Protein: 6g

Brown Rice with Asparagus and Walnuts

SERVES 4 • PREP TIME: 5 MINUTES • COOK TIME: 55 MINUTES

This nutritious side dish incorporates foods rich in nutrients recommended on the DASH diet. Brown rice is a whole grain and provides your body with long-lasting energy from its abundance of vitamins, minerals, and fiber. Asparagus, a natural diuretic, boosts the potassium content, and walnuts add a delicious taste as well as healthy omega-3 fats. Serve alongside your favorite lean protein.

1 tablespoon olive oil

½ cup finely chopped onion

2 garlic cloves, minced

½ cup brown rice

1 cup water

Freshly ground black pepper

1 cup chopped thin asparagus (1-inch pieces)

¼ cup walnuts, chopped

1. In a medium saucepan, heat the olive oil over medium-high heat. Add the onion and garlic, and cook for 3 to 5 minutes, or until the vegetables are tender. Add the rice, and, stirring constantly, cook for another 2 to 3 minutes.

2. Add the water, bring to a boil, and cook uncovered for 3 minutes. Lower the heat, and season with the black pepper. Cover and simmer for 30 minutes.

3. Gently stir in the asparagus, re-cover, and continue simmering for 5 to 10 minutes, or until the liquid is absorbed.

4. Gently stir in the walnuts, cover the saucepan, and set aside for 5 minutes.

5. Serve immediately.

SUBSTITUTION TIP For a dish with more protein, vitamins, minerals, and fiber, add 1 (15-ounce) can of drained and rinsed chickpeas when you add the asparagus. Adding the beans will increase the calorie count.

Nutrition (per serving) Calories: 151; Total Fat: 9g; Saturated Fat: 1g; Cholesterol: 0mg; Sodium: 2mg; Potassium: 200mg; Magnesium: 40mg; Total Carbohydrates: 16g; Fiber: 3g; Sugars: 0g; Protein: 3g

Rosemary Roasted Beets and Carrots

SERVES 4 • PREP TIME: 5 MINUTES • COOK TIME: 35 MINUTES

Sweet and earthy beets are packed with a surprising number of heart-health benefits and should enjoy a much-deserved place in your DASH diet. Many of the benefits come from the naturally occurring nitrates in beets, which are converted to nitric oxide in your body. Nitric oxide improves blood flow and lowers blood pressure. When roasted, beets become syrupy-tasting and utterly delicious.

1½ pounds beets, peeled and cut into ½-inch wedges

1 pound carrots, scrubbed and cut into 2-inch pieces

⅓ cup red wine vinegar

2 tablespoons olive oil

2 fresh rosemary sprigs

¼ teaspoon freshly ground black pepper

1. Preheat the oven to 450°F.

2. In a large bowl, combine all of the ingredients, and toss to evenly coat the vegetables.

3. Spread the vegetables on a rimmed baking sheet and roast, tossing once, for 30 to 35 minutes, or until the vegetables are tender.

4. Serve immediately.

SUBSTITUTION TIP In place of the carrots, you can use other root vegetables that also pair well with beets, including turnips, parsnips, butternut squash, yams or sweet potatoes, red potatoes, and rutabaga.

Nutrition (per serving) Calories: 180; Total Fat: 8g; Saturated Fat: 1g; Cholesterol: 0mg; Sodium: 211mg; Potassium: 932mg; Magnesium: 53mg; Total Carbohydrates: 27g; Fiber: 8g; Sugars: 17g; Protein: 4g

Creamed Swiss Chard

SERVES 4 • PREP TIME: 5 MINUTES • COOK TIME: 5 MINUTES

Available year-round, Swiss chard is among the most tender and sweetest of the cooking greens. Like all dark leafy greens, Swiss chard is a nutritional powerhouse and a rich source of blood pressure–lowering minerals, including calcium, magnesium, and potassium. Ready in just minutes, low-fat milk contributes a rich flavor and added calcium to this healthy DASH side dish.

1½ tablespoons olive oil

1½ tablespoons unbleached plain flour

3 garlic cloves, minced

1 cup nonfat or low-fat milk

2 pounds Swiss chard, washed, stemmed, and cut crosswise into ½-inch-wide strips

½ teaspoon freshly ground black pepper

1. In a large frying pan, heat the olive oil over medium heat. Whisk in the flour to make a smooth paste. Continue whisking, add the garlic, and cook for another 30 seconds. Whisk in the milk and cook for 2 to 3 minutes, or until the mixture thickens slightly.

2. Add the Swiss chard and stir to coat well. Cover and cook just until tender, about 2 minutes. Season with the black pepper.

3. Serve immediately.

SUBSTITUTION TIP Low-fat soy milk can be used in place of nonfat or low-fat dairy milk. The benefit of this substitution is the elimination of dietary cholesterol. Soy milk is fortified with calcium and most brands contain higher levels than cow's milk.

Nutrition (per serving) Calories: 128; Total Fat: 6g; Saturated Fat: 1g; Cholesterol: 1mg; Sodium: 432mg; Potassium: 1,352mg; Magnesium: 204mg; Total Carbohydrates: 14g; Fiber: 5g; Sugars: 6g; Protein: 7g

Lemon-Parmesan Broccoli

SERVES 4 • PREP TIME: 5 MINUTES • COOK TIME: 6 MINUTES

Being a cruciferous vegetable, broccoli is a rich source of vitamins, minerals, and antioxidants, and contains valuable plant nutrients shown to be protective against cancer. Low in calories and a good source of potassium, magnesium, calcium, and fiber, this quick-and-easy recipe makes it simple to incorporate broccoli into your DASH diet.

4 cups broccoli florets

1½ tablespoons olive oil

2 garlic cloves, minced

1 teaspoon freshly squeezed lemon juice

2 tablespoons shaved fresh Parmesan cheese

1. In a pot fitted with a steamer basket, arrange the broccoli florets, and cover. Steam for 4 minutes, or until the broccoli is crisp-tender. Transfer to a large bowl.

2. Heat a small skillet over medium-high heat. Add the olive oil and garlic. Cook for 2 minutes, or until the garlic is fragrant.

3. Pour the oil mixture and lemon juice over the broccoli. Toss to coat. Sprinkle with the cheese.

4. Serve immediately.

SUBSTITUTION TIP For a variation of this recipe, add 1 tablespoon of minced shallot and 1 teaspoon of dried thyme to the oil and garlic in step 2, and replace the cheese with 2 tablespoons of pine nuts.

Nutrition (per serving) Calories: 82; Total Fat: 6g; Saturated Fat: 1g; Cholesterol: 3mg; Sodium: 67mg; Potassium: 292mg; Magnesium: 24mg; Total Carbohydrates: 5g; Fiber: 3g; Sugars: 0g; Protein: 4g

Chocolate Mint "Ice Cream"

SERVES 4 • PREP TIME: 10 MINUTES

Keeping sugar intake to a minimum while you are following the DASH diet doesn't mean you can't have any treats. While this recipe isn't technically ice cream, it's amazing how much it seems like the real thing. It's made with three simple ingredients: bananas, cocoa powder, and peppermint extract. And the best part is, it's loaded with potassium, fiber, and beneficial plant antioxidants, making it a perfect fit for DASH.

3 bananas, sliced and frozen

4 tablespoons unsweetened cocoa powder

½ teaspoon peppermint extract

2 to 3 tablespoons nonfat or low-fat milk (optional)

1. Remove the frozen bananas from the freezer and let stand for about 5 minutes.

2. Add the banana, cocoa, and peppermint extract to a food processor and pulse until the banana slices are finely chopped. Then purée until the mixture resembles soft-serve ice cream, adding the milk (if using).

INGREDIENT TIP If the "ice cream" becomes too soft after puréeing, place it in the freezer for several minutes to firm up slightly before serving. Freeze any leftover amount, and let it stand at room temperature for 5 to 10 minutes before serving.

Nutrition (per serving) Calories: 92; Total Fat: 1g; Saturated Fat: 1g; Cholesterol: 0mg; Sodium: 2mg; Potassium: 400mg; Magnesium: 53mg; Total Carbohydrates: 23g; Fiber: 4g; Sugars: 11g; Protein: 2g

Grilled Banana Split Bowl

SERVES 2 • PREP TIME: 10 MINUTES

Including plenty of produce in your diet is one of the key parts of DASH, and one of the best choices for fruit is the potassium-rich banana. Inspired by a banana-split dessert, this grilled–banana split bowl kicks the nutrition up a notch by adding protein-rich Greek yogurt in place of high-fat, sugar-loaded ice cream. If you are in a rush, you can skip the grilling, but it gives the bananas added taste.

¾ cup plain low-fat Greek yogurt

2 tablespoons low-sugar strawberry jam

½ teaspoon vanilla extract

1 large banana, unpeeled and halved lengthwise

½ teaspoon olive oil

⅓ cup diced pineapple (fresh or canned, drained)

1 tablespoon sliced almonds

½ cup diced fresh strawberries

1. Heat a grill pan or grill to medium.

2. In a small bowl, whisk together the yogurt, jam, and vanilla extract until well combined. Set aside.

3. Brush or rub the cut side of the banana halves with the olive oil. Grill the banana halves, cut-side down, over direct medium heat for 6 to 7 minutes, or until caramelized. Then grill the peel side of the banana halves until heated through, about 1 minute. Gently remove the peels.

4. Place one grilled banana half in each of two bowls and top each half with half of the yogurt-jam mixture, pineapple, almonds, and strawberries.

5. Serve immediately.

SUBSTITUTION TIP You can customize this recipe to suit your personal tastes and vary the flavor of jam, swap the pineapple and strawberries for in-season fruit, and replace the sliced almonds with any other unsalted nut such as walnuts, peanuts, or cashews.

Nutrition (per serving) Calories: 193; Total Fat: 5g; Saturated Fat: 1g; Cholesterol: 5mg; Sodium: 37mg; Potassium: 363mg; Magnesium: 32mg; Total Carbohydrates: 31g; Fiber: 4g; Sugars: 17g; Protein: 10g

Peanut Butter Rice Pudding

SERVES 4 • PREP TIME: 5 MINUTES • COOK TIME: 40 MINUTES

High in calcium, fiber, and protein, peanut butter–rice pudding is an easy and nutritious DASH-friendly dessert that can be made with just a few ingredients. Using no difficult cooking techniques, this sweet and satisfying dessert helps you meet your recommended servings for whole grains, dairy, and legumes.

1 cup uncooked brown rice

2½ cups nonfat milk

¼ cup unsalted natural peanut butter

⅔ cup water

2 teaspoons pure vanilla extract

1 tablespoon honey (more or less to taste)

1. In a medium saucepan, combine the rice and milk, and bring to a boil.

2. Lower to a simmer and cover. Simmer, covered, for 20 to 40 minutes, or until rice is thick and fluffy. (Length of time depends on the variety of brown rice used.)

3. Stir in the peanut butter and water and return to a boil. Remove from the heat. Allow to sit, covered, for 15 to 20 minutes, or until the water is absorbed.

4. Stir in the vanilla and honey.

5. Enjoy warm or cold.

SUBSTITUTION TIP For a flavor variation, stir in 1 tablespoon of chocolate chips or low-sugar jam, or ¼ cup of fresh berries. You can also use your favorite nut butter in place of peanut butter, such as almond butter, cashew butter, pumpkin-seed butter, or others.

Nutrition (per serving) Calories: 262; Total Fat: 9g; Saturated Fat: 2g; Cholesterol: 2mg; Sodium: 92mg; Potassium: 226mg; Magnesium: 53mg; Total Carbohydrates: 35g; Fiber: 3g; Sugars: 10g; Protein: 9g

Chocolate-Covered Strawberry Smoothie

SERVES 2 • PREP TIME: 5 MINUTES

Thick and creamy smoothies make extremely satisfying snacks or desserts, dazzling your taste buds while providing your body with a nutritious mix of ingredients. Both strawberries and cocoa have been studied for their blood pressure–lowering effects due to their high levels of antioxidants. Blended with high-protein Greek yogurt, this decadent-tasting smoothie is a perfect fit for your DASH eating plan.

1 to 2 cups ice

1 cup nonfat or low-fat milk

¾ cup plain nonfat or low-fat Greek yogurt

1 cup frozen strawberries

1 frozen banana, peeled and sliced

2 tablespoons unsweetened cocoa powder

½ teaspoon vanilla extract

1 teaspoon honey (optional)

1. In a blender, combine all of the ingredients, and blend until smooth.

2. Pour into two tall glasses and enjoy immediately.

SUBSTITUTION TIP You can substitute cacao in place of cocoa in this recipe. Cacao is the purest form of chocolate you can consume, which means it is raw and less processed than cocoa. While both have about the same levels of antioxidants, cacao has higher levels of magnesium.

Nutrition (per serving) Calories: 181; Total Fat: 1g; Saturated Fat: 1g; Cholesterol: 6mg; Sodium: 98mg; Potassium: 788mg; Magnesium: 68mg; Total Carbohydrates: 33g; Fiber: 5g; Sugars: 21g; Protein: 15g

Simple Sweet Potato Brownies

MAKES 12 BROWNIES • PREP TIME: 5 MINUTES • COOK TIME: 20 MINUTES

Just a handful of ingredients are needed to prepare these rich, fudgy, and extremely moist chocolate brownies. Using nutrient-rich sweet potato as the base, these flourless brownies are free of refined sugar. They are high in fiber, vitamins A and C, potassium, and plant antioxidants. This quick-and-easy snack recipe will satisfy your sweet tooth in a healthy way.

½ cup unsalted smooth nut butter (peanut, almond, cashew)

2 tablespoons maple syrup

1 cup cooked mashed sweet potato

½ teaspoon vanilla extract

½ teaspoon ground cinnamon

¼ cup unsweetened cocoa powder

1. Preheat the oven to 350°F. Grease a brownie pan or loaf pan and set aside.

2. In a small microwave-safe bowl or on the stovetop, melt together the nut butter and maple syrup.

3. In a large mixing bowl, combine the melted-nut butter mixture, mashed sweet potato, vanilla extract, cinnamon, and cocoa powder. Mix until well combined.

4. Pour the mixture into the pan and bake for about 20 minutes, or until cooked through.

5. Remove from the oven and allow to cool completely before slicing and serving.

INGREDIENT TIP These brownies are best kept in the refrigerator and eaten when completely cooled, but they also freeze well. Simply wrap them tightly in freezer wrap and enjoy within a month.

Nutrition (1 brownie) Calories: 94; Total Fat: 6g; Saturated Fat: 1g; Cholesterol: 0mg; Sodium: 37mg; Potassium: 55mg; Magnesium: 12mg; Total Carbohydrates: 9g; Fiber: 2g; Sugars: 3g; Protein: 3g

Banana-Chocolate Chip Muffins

MAKES 12 MUFFINS • PREP TIME: 10 MINUTES • COOK TIME: 20 TO 25 MINUTES

These healthy, potassium- and protein-rich banana muffins are quick to prepare and make a nutritious and delicious snack. This recipe uses whole-wheat flour, which is a fiber-rich whole grain, Greek yogurt in place of butter to keep the muffins moist and to provide protein to keep you feeling full, honey in place of sugar, and chocolate chips for a bit of indulgence.

1½ cups whole-wheat pastry flour

1 teaspoon baking soda

¼ teaspoon salt

3 very ripe bananas

2 tablespoons honey

1 teaspoon vanilla extract

1 egg

½ cup plain nonfat Greek yogurt

1 tablespoon nonfat milk

½ cup chocolate chips

1. Preheat the oven to 350°F. Spray a 12-cup muffin tin with nonstick cooking spray.

2. In a medium bowl, whisk together the flour, baking soda, and salt.

3. In a blender, combine the bananas, honey, vanilla, egg, yogurt, and milk. Blend on high for 1 minute or until well combined, smooth, and creamy.

4. Add the wet ingredients to the dry ingredients, and mix until just combined. Gently fold in the chocolate chips.

5. Divide the batter evenly among the muffin tins and bake for 20 to 25 minutes, or until a toothpick inserted in the center comes out clean. Let the muffins cool in the pan for 5 minutes, then transfer to a wire rack to finish cooling.

6. Enjoy warm or cool. Freeze leftovers in an airtight container for up to 3 months.

INGREDIENT TIP Whole-wheat pastry flour is lighter than regular whole-wheat flour and is the preferred type for making quick breads and muffins. Your muffins will turn out fine if all you have is regular whole-wheat flour; they will just be a bit denser.

Nutrition (1 muffin) Calories: 137; Total Fat: 4g; Saturated Fat: 2g; Cholesterol: 19mg; Sodium: 171mg; Potassium: 169mg; Magnesium: 20mg; Total Carbohydrates: 25g; Fiber: 2g; Sugars: 12g; Protein: 4g

Cilantro-Strawberry Salsa, page 148

CHAPTER

9

Broths, Condiments & Sauces

Cilantro-Strawberry Salsa

YIELD: 4 CUPS • PREP TIME: 10 MINUTES

This tasty salsa has a hidden blood pressure–lowering ingredient: fresh strawberries. Combined with traditional salsa ingredients, including fresh tomatoes, lime, and garlic, this sweet berry provides a nice flavor contrast, making this a suitable topping for Mexican dishes or as a dip for whole-grain tortilla chips.

2 medium fresh tomatoes, stems removed and diced

2 scallions, chopped

2 garlic cloves, minced

1 jalapeño pepper, stems, ribs, and seeds removed, finely diced

Juice of 1 lime

1 cup diced fresh strawberries

½ cup chopped fresh cilantro

Pinch oregano

Pinch cumin

1. In a medium mixing bowl, combine all of the ingredients, and stir gently.

2. Serve immediately.

Nutrition (½ cup) Calories: 23; Total Fat: 0g; Saturated Fat: 0g; Cholesterol: 0mg; Sodium: 5mg; Potassium: 169mg; Magnesium: 8mg; Total Carbohydrates: 5g; Fiber: 1g; Sugars: 2g; Protein: 1g

Creamy Avocado Dressing

YIELD: 1 CUP • PREP TIME: 5 MINUTES

Creamy salad dressings are often loaded with calories, unhealthy fats, and sodium. Even a tablespoon or two on a salad can easily pack on at least a hundred calories. Luckily, with this healthier alternative to creamy dressing, you can enjoy a rich taste on your vegetables with the added nutritional benefits of avocado for your heart.

1 avocado, peeled and seeded

2 garlic cloves, minced

¼ cup roughly chopped fresh cilantro

¼ cup low-fat or nonfat plain Greek yogurt

2 tablespoons freshly squeezed lime or lemon juice

2 tablespoons olive oil

¼ teaspoon freshly ground black pepper

⅓ cup water

1. In a blender or food processor, combine all of the ingredients, with the exception of the water. Blend or process until smooth, stopping to scrape down the sides a few times.

2. Thin the dressing out with the water a little at a time until it reaches the desired consistency.

3. Keep the dressing in an airtight container in the refrigerator for up to one week.

SUBSTITUTION TIP You can use white wine vinegar in place of the lemon or lime juice. You can also use whatever herbs and spices you desire.

Nutrition (1 tablespoon) Calories: 36; Total Fat: 3g; Saturated Fat: 1g; Cholesterol: 0mg; Sodium: 3mg; Potassium: 64mg; Magnesium: 32mg; Total Carbohydrates: 1g; Fiber: 1g; Sugars: 0g; Protein: 1g

Italian Salad Dressing

YIELD: ½ CUP • PREP TIME: 5 MINUTES

This budget-friendly, quick, and easy homemade salad dressing is full of flavor and can be made in minutes using a handful of pantry staples. With no added salt and heart-healthy olive oil, you can enjoy this Italian-style dressing on your favorite salad.

4 tablespoons olive oil

3 tablespoons red wine vinegar

2 tablespoons freshly squeezed lemon juice

3 teaspoons Dijon mustard

2 cloves garlic, minced

2 teaspoons dried basil

1 teaspoon dried parsley

¼ teaspoon dried oregano

¼ teaspoon crushed red pepper flakes

1. Combine all of the ingredients in a jar. Cover tightly with a screw cap, and shake to mix.

2. Keep the dressing in an airtight container in the refrigerator for up to one week.

INGREDIENT TIP When using olive oil as a condiment, consider investing in high-quality extra-virgin olive oil. Extra-virgin olive oil is the highest grade of olive oil and is made without the use of chemicals or excessive heat.

Nutrition (1 tablespoon) Calories: 55; Total Fat: 6g; Saturated Fat: 1g; Cholesterol: 0mg; Sodium: 40mg; Potassium: 5mg; Magnesium: 0mg; Total Carbohydrates: 0g; Fiber: 0g; Sugars: 0g; Protein: 0g

Tzatziki Sauce

YIELD: 2 CUPS • PREP TIME: 5 MINUTES

Tzatziki is a Greek-yogurt sauce traditionally used on kebabs, falafel, and barbecued meats. You can also use it as a dip for veggies or pita chips, or as a salad dressing. Nothing beats the freshness and taste of homemade dips, especially when they are this easy to make. High in calcium, tzatziki fits perfectly into your DASH eating plan.

1 medium English cucumber, seeded

1½ cups plain low-fat Greek yogurt

2 small garlic cloves, minced

1 teaspoon freshly squeezed lemon juice

Dash freshly ground black pepper

2 tablespoons finely chopped fresh mint or dill

1. Coarsely grate the cucumber into a medium bowl, and drain off the excess liquid.

2. Add the yogurt, garlic, lemon juice, black pepper, and mint or dill. Mix well.

3. Refrigerate to chill for about an hour before serving.

INGREDIENT TIP If you have the time, strain the yogurt using a metal strainer or coffee filter for a few hours to remove as much liquid as possible. This produces a thicker, more traditional tzatziki sauce.

Nutrition (1 tablespoon) Calories: 10; Total Fat: 0g; Saturated Fat: 0g; Cholesterol: 1mg; Sodium: 4mg; Potassium: 1mg; Magnesium: 0mg; Total Carbohydrates: 1g; Fiber: 0g; Sugars: 1g; Protein: 1g

Simple Tomato Sauce

YIELD: 4 CUPS • PREP TIME: 5 MINUTES • COOK TIME: 1 HOUR

Processed tomato and spaghetti sauces generally contain far too much sodium for the DASH diet. Many also contain added fats and fillers that provide no nutritional benefit. You can skip the processed sauce, save some money, and get the benefit of more vitamins, minerals, and fiber by making your own.

1 tablespoon olive oil

1 cup minced
yellow onion

4 garlic cloves, minced

1 (28-ounce) can
no-salt crushed
tomatoes

¼ cup water

2 tablespoons no-salt
added tomato paste

2 tablespoons honey

2 tablespoons oregano

1 tablespoon basil

½ teaspoon crushed
red pepper flakes

1. In a large pot over medium heat, heat the olive oil. Add the onion and garlic and cook for 3 to 5 minutes, or until tender. Reduce the heat to low.

2. Add the remaining ingredients, and cover. Cook over low heat for 50 to 60 minutes.

3. Taste to adjust seasonings.

4. Serve hot as you would store-bought tomato sauce. Store any leftovers in an airtight container in the refrigerator for up to one week.

INGREDIENT TIP If you decide to add salt to a dish for flavor, keep in mind that a dash of salt is a scant ⅛ teaspoon, which contains 250 mg of sodium. If you do add it, be sure to include it in your sodium count for the day.

Nutrition (½ cup) Calories: 71; Total Fat: 2g; Saturated Fat: 0g; Cholesterol: 0mg; Sodium: 16mg; Potassium: 333mg; Magnesium: 20mg; Total Carbohydrates: 13g; Fiber: 2g; Sugars: 5g; Protein: 2g

Five-Spice Mango Stir-Fry Sauce

YIELD: 1 CUP • PREP TIME: 5 MINUTES

Stir-fry sauces are typically very high in sodium, even for the very small amounts called for in most recipes. It is really easy to make a homemade sauce that's much healthier and lower in sodium. This recipe uses the sweet-tasting, potassium-rich mango to create a delicious sauce that will jazz up your next stir-fry.

1 cup mango cubes

3 tablespoons brown sugar

2 teaspoons freshly squeezed lime juice

1 teaspoon sesame oil

1 tablespoon water

2 garlic cloves

½ teaspoon Chinese 5-spice powder

¼ teaspoon red pepper flakes

1. In a blender, combine all of the ingredients, and blend until smooth.

2. Use immediately or store in the refrigerator in an airtight container for two to three days, or in the freezer for up to three months.

SERVING TIP In a large frying pan or wok, toss the sauce with your choice of 4 to 6 ounces of cooked protein for 1 minute, or until heated through. Add 1 to 2 cups of cooked veggies, and toss to coat. Serve over brown rice.

Nutrition (¼ cup) Calories: 64; Total Fat: 1g; Saturated Fat: 0g; Cholesterol: 0mg; Sodium: 4mg; Potassium: 94mg; Magnesium: 6mg; Total Carbohydrates: 17g; Fiber: 1g; Sugars: 15g; Protein: 0g

Potato Vegetable Broth

YIELD: 10 CUPS • PREP TIME: 15 MINUTE • COOK TIME: 30 MINUTES

Stocks and broths are kitchen staples that amp up the flavor of your favorite recipes. While you can easily purchase broth at the supermarket, processed varieties contain a host of additives you may not want in your diet. Making your own stock is cheap, and it really is easy to do. Plus, it cuts down on food waste and is generally higher in nutrients than what you can purchase. This broth has a rich taste from potatoes and leeks.

2 pounds potatoes, scrubbed, peeled, and cut into 1-inch pieces

4 large leeks, white parts only, split, well-rinsed, and sliced

2 medium carrots, scrubbed and cut into 1-inch pieces

½ teaspoon freshly ground black pepper

1 bay leaf

1 teaspoon dried thyme

1. In a heavy-bottomed stockpot, combine all of the ingredients. Add about 8 cups of water or more as needed to completely cover the vegetables.

2. Bring to a boil, reduce heat, cover, and simmer for 30 minutes.

3. Pass the broth through a large sieve or colander, pressing on the vegetables to extract as much juice as possible. Discard the vegetable pulp.

4. Store in the refrigerator in an airtight container for four to five days. Use it generously as needed in your favorite recipes.

INGREDIENT TIP If you won't be using all of your broth within four to five days, freeze it in an airtight container for four to six months.

Nutrition (1 cup) Calories: 10; Total Fat: 0g; Saturated Fat: 0g; Cholesterol: 0mg; Sodium: 29mg; Potassium: 469mg; Magnesium: 32mg; Total Carbohydrates: 2g; Fiber: 0g; Sugars: 0g; Protein: 1g

Homemade Chicken Broth

YIELD: 8 CUPS • PREP TIME: 15 MINUTES • COOK TIME: 2 HOURS

Nothing is more soothing or comforting than homemade chicken broth. Easy to make and economical, homemade broth delivers maximum flavor while contributing minimal calories. Freeze excess broth in recipe-ready amounts so you have some on hand for quick soups.

4 quarts cold water

1 (3-pound) whole chicken (or chicken parts, such as wings and breasts)

4 celery stalks with leaves, trimmed and cut into 2-inch pieces

4 medium carrots, peeled and cut into 2-inch pieces

1 medium onion, peeled and quartered

1 medium potato, peeled and quartered

6 garlic cloves

1 small bunch parsley

1 teaspoon dried thyme

2 bay leaves

1. In a large stockpot, combine all of the ingredients, and bring to a boil over medium-high heat. Reduce the heat to medium-low and simmer, partially covered, until the chicken is falling apart, about 2 hours.

2. Strain the broth through a large sieve or colander into a large bowl. Use a wooden spoon to press on the solids to extract as much of the broth as possible. Save the chicken meat if desired or discard along with the vegetable pulp and bones.

3. Allow the broth to cool in the bowl or divide the broth among several shallow containers to cool it quickly.

4. Cover loosely and refrigerate overnight. Use a spoon to remove the fat that congeals on the surface before using.

INGREDIENT TIP Store the broth in an airtight container in the refrigerator for up to two days, or freeze it for up to three months.

Nutrition (1 cup) Calories: 86; Total Fat: 3g; Saturated Fat: 1g; Cholesterol: 7mg; Sodium: 50mg; Potassium: 252mg; Magnesium: 10mg; Total Carbohydrates: 9g; Fiber: 0g; Sugars: 1g; Protein: 6g

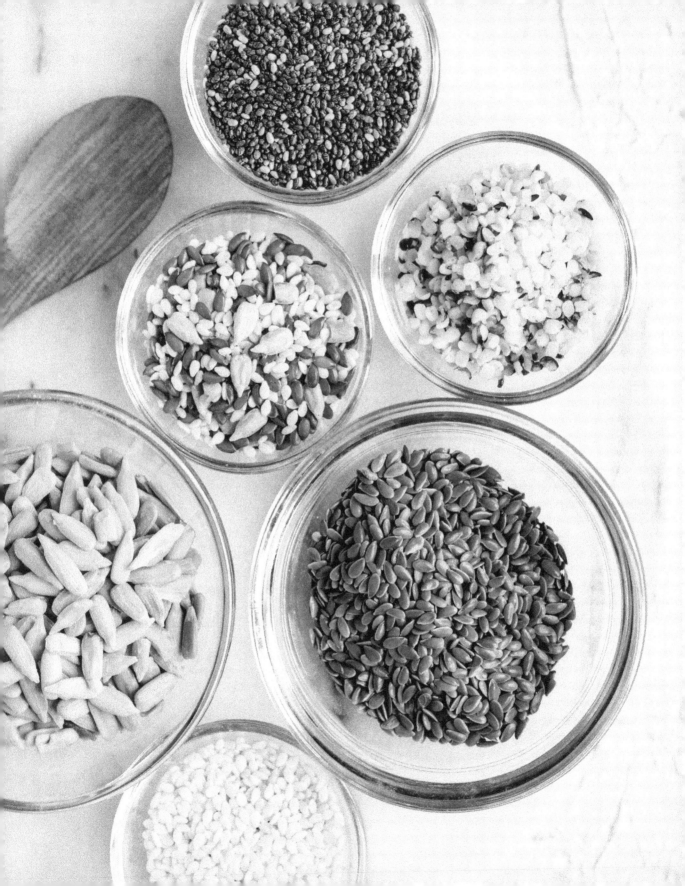

TIPS FOR EATING OUT

Healthy Restaurant Choices

You can order heart-healthy options at any restaurant; you just have to be strategic. Here are some ordering tips to use when eating out:

- Request that your food be prepared without salt or salty seasonings.
- Keep condiments on the side.
- Watch your liquid calories and choose water as your beverage.
- Choose baked, broiled, and grilled entrées and skip the fried.
- Skip heavy cream sauces and choose marinara over Alfredo-type sauces.
- Go for fish, chicken, and vegetarian dishes instead of red meat.
- Watch portion sizes and fill half your plate with vegetables.
- Go easy on the bread and chips.

Healthy Mexican tips and picks: Limit your intake of chips and start with tortilla soup instead. Opt for vegetable- and bean-filled soft tacos, tamales, and burritos over fried items. Fajitas are a good choice because you can control the portions since the meat, veggies, toppings, and tortillas are all served separately. Ask for less cheese, sour cream, and guacamole.

Healthy Chinese tips and picks: Skip the soup and noodles, and choose steamed dishes with sauce on the side. Choose entrées that come with a lot of vegetables like Moo Goo Gai Pan. Ask for brown rice instead of white.

Healthy pizza tips and picks: Choose a thin-crust pizza over a thick-crust or stuffed. Ask for extra veggies and light cheese instead of adding meat options. Start with a salad with dressing on the side, and choose water as your beverage.

Heart-Healthy Snacks

Reach for snacks that include two to three food groups. Combining fruits and vegetables with whole grains, lean proteins, and healthy fats makes a snack that is satisfying and filling. Try one of these 20 snacks that are flavorful, satisfying, and easy to grab and go:

1. Apple with unsalted nut butter
2. Edamame
3. Nonfat or low-fat regular yogurt or Greek yogurt with fruit
4. Whole-grain English muffin topped with tomatoes and low-fat mozzarella cheese
5. Hummus and vegetable sticks
6. Low-fat string cheese and fruit
7. Hardboiled egg and fruit
8. 1 ounce of unsalted nuts and veggie sticks
9. Bean dip and whole-grain pita chips
10. Whole-grain bread with nut butter
11. Unbuttered, unsalted popcorn
12. Nonfat or low-fat milk or plain soy milk
13. Roasted chickpeas
14. Rice cakes with nut butter
15. Canned tuna or salmon with whole-grain crackers
16. Nonfat or low-fat cottage cheese and tomatoes
17. Small cup of low-sodium bean soup
18. Bowl of whole-grain cereal with low-fat milk
19. Dried-fruit and nut mix
20. Yogurt smoothie

MEASUREMENT CONVERSIONS

Volume Equivalents (Dry)

US STANDARD	METRIC (APPROX.)
⅛ teaspoon	0.5 mL
¼ teaspoon	1 mL
½ teaspoon	2 mL
¾ teaspoon	4 mL
1 teaspoon	5 mL
1 tablespoon	15 mL
¼ cup	59 mL
⅓ cup	79 mL
½ cup	118 mL
⅔ cup	156 mL
¾ cup	177 mL
1 cup	235 mL
2 cups or 1 pint	475 mL
3 cups	700 mL
4 cups or 1 quart	1 L
½ gallon	2 L
1 gallon	4 L

Volume Equivalents (Liquid)

US STANDARD	US STANDARD (OUNCES)	METRIC (APPROX.)
2 tablespoons	1 fl. oz.	30 mL
¼ cup	2 fl. oz.	60 mL
½ cup	4 fl. oz.	120 mL
1 cup	8 fl. oz.	240 mL
1½ cups	12 fl. oz.	355 mL
2 cups or 1 pint	16 fl. oz.	475 mL
4 cups or 1 quart	32 fl. oz.	1 L
1 gallon	128 fl. oz.	4 L

Oven Temperatures

FAHRENHEIT (F)	CELSIUS (C) (APPROX.)
250°F	120°C
300°F	150°C
325°F	165°C
350°F	180°C
375°F	190°C
400°F	200°C
425°F	220°C
450°F	230°C

Weight Equivalents

US STANDARD	METRIC (APPROX.)
½ ounce	15 g
1 ounce	30 g
2 ounces	60 g
4 ounces	115 g
8 ounces	225 g
12 ounces	340 g
16 ounces or 1 pound	455 g

THE DIRTY DOZEN AND THE CLEAN FIFTEEN

A nonprofit and environmental organization called Environmental Working Group (EWG) looks at data supplied by the US Department of Agriculture (USDA) and the Food and Drug Administration (FDA) about pesticide residues and compiles a list each year of the best and worst pesticide loads found in commercial crops. The Dirty Dozen list advises which fruits and vegetables you should always buy organic. The Clean Fifteen list lets you know which produce is considered safe enough, when grown conventionally, to allow you to skip the organics. This does not mean that the Clean Fifteen produce is pesticide-free, though, so wash these fruits and vegetables thoroughly.

These lists change every year, so make sure you look up the most recent before you fill your shopping cart. You'll find the most recent lists as well as a guide to pesticides in produce at www.EWG.org/FoodNews.

2017 Dirty Dozen

Apples	Spinach
Celery	Strawberries
Cherry tomatoes	Sweet bell peppers
Cucumbers	In addition to the Dirty Dozen, the EWG added two foods contaminated with highly toxic organophosphate insecticides:
Grapes	
Nectarines	
Peaches	
Potatoes	
Snap peas	Hot peppers
	Kale/Collard greens

2017 Clean Fifteen

Asparagus	Onions
Avocados	Papayas
Cabbage	Pineapples
Cantaloupe	Sweet corn
Cauliflower	Sweet peas (frozen)
Eggplant	Sweet potatoes
Grapefruit	
Kiwis	
Mangoes	

REFERENCES

American Heart Association. "High Blood Pressure Homepage." Accessed May 17, 2017. www.heart.org/HEARTORG/Conditions/HighBloodPressure /High-Blood-Pressure-or-Hypertension_UCM_002020_SubHomePage.jsp.

American Heart Association. "What About High Blood Pressure and African Americans?" American Heart Association. Accessed May 17, 2017. www.heart.org/idc/groups/heart-public/@wcm/@hcm/documents/downloadable /ucm_300463.pdf.doi: 10.2337/dc13-2042.

Evert, Alison B., Jackie L. Boucher, Marjorie Cypress, Stephanie A. Dunbar, Marion J. Franz, Elizabeth J. Mayer-Davis, and Joshua J. Neumiller, et al. "Nutrition Therapy Recommendations for the Management of Adults with Diabetes." *Diabetes Care* Vol 36 No. 11 (2013): 3821-3842.

Health.gov. "2015–2020 Dietary Guidelines for Americans." Office of Disease Prevention and Health Promotion. Accessed May 17, 2017. www.health.gov /dietaryguidelines/2015.

National Heart, Lung, and Blood Institute. "DASH Eating Plan." September 16, 2015. Accessed May 17, 2017. www.nhlbi.nih.gov/health/health-topics/topics/dash.

National Institute of Diabetes and Digestive and Kidney Diseases. "High Blood Pressure & Kidney Disease." September 2014. Accessed May 17, 2017. www.niddk.nih.gov/health-information/kidney-disease/chronic-kidney-disease -ckd/high-blood-pressure.

National Institutes of Health. "Magnesium." February 11, 2016. Accessed June 21, 2017. www.ods.od.nih.gov/factsheets/Magnesium-HealthProfessional.

Neff, Kristin. "Self-Compassion." Accessed June 21, 2017. www.self-compassion.org.

Sacks, Frank M., Alice Lichtenstein, Linda Van Horn, William Harris, Penny Kris-Etherton, and Mary Winston. "Soy Protein, Isoflavones, and Cardiovascular Health." *Circulation* 113, Issue 7 (February 2006): 1034-1044. circ.ahajournals.org/content/113/7/1034.

U.S. News and World Report. "Best Diets Overall." U.S. News. Accessed June 21, 2017. health.usnews.com/best-diet/best-diets-overall.

RESOURCES

The Mayo Clinic website provides an in-depth description of the DASH diet as well as a two-day sample DASH diet menu:

- DASH Diet: Healthy Eating to Lower Your Blood Pressure. www.mayoclinic.org/healthy-lifestyle/nutrition-and-healthy-eating/in-depth /dash-diet/art-20048456

- Sample menus for the DASH diet. www.mayoclinic.org/healthy-lifestyle/nutrition-and-healthy-eating/in-depth /dash-diet/art-20047110?pg=1

The National Heart, Lung, and Blood Institute promotes the DASH diet. You will find pages of useful information on their website:

- DASH Eating Plan. National Heart, Lung, and Blood Institute. www.nhlbi.nih.gov /health/health-topics/topics/dash

The USDA Dietary Guidelines for Americans recommends the DASH eating plan as a healthy eating pattern to follow. On this site you will find information on food groups, food-group servings, and related healthy lifestyle information:

- Health.gov. 2015-2020 Dietary Guidelines for Americans. www.health.gov /dietaryguidelines/2015

The Academy of Nutrition and Dietetics website has articles and nutrition information for consumers on heart and cardiovascular health:

- Heart and Cardiovascular Health. Academy of Nutrition and Dietetics. www.eatright.org/resources/health/wellness/heart-and-cardiovascular-health

The Mediterranean Diet shares many similarities with the DASH diet. To learn more visit:

- Mediterranean Diet: A Heart Healthy Eating Plan. Mayo Clinic. www.mayoclinic.org/healthy-lifestyle/nutrition-and-healthy-eating/in-depth /mediterranean-diet/art-20047801

The Centers for Disease Control and Prevention hosts a site called Million Hearts where you can find meal plans and recipes designed for heart health:

- Millions Hearts. Centers for Disease Control and Prevention. millionhearts.hhs.gov/learn-prevent/recipes.html

For a description of symptoms, heart-healthy guidelines, and other tools, visit:

- Nutrition, Diet & Your Health. Seconds Count.org. www.secondscount.org /healthy-living/heart-healthy-nutrition-diet#.WDtIAqIrJ-U

The American Heart Association website has heart-healthy recipes and nutrition information geared toward the consumer:

- The American Heart Association. Heart-Healthy Recipes. recipes.heart.org /?gclid=CObGs4HsydACFYM2gQodtaoIrA
- The American Heart Association. Nutrition. www.heart.org/HEARTORG /HealthyLiving/HealthyEating/Nutrition/Nutrition_UCM_310436 _SubHomePage.jsp

The Oregon Dairy Council website has a wealth of resources, recipes, and tools to help you get started on following the DASH diet:

- www.dashdietoregon.org

RECIPE INDEX

INDEX

ABOUT THE AUTHOR

JENNIFER KOSLO is a Registered Dietitian Nutritionist (RDN), Board Certified Specialist in Sports Dietetics (CSSD), Licensed Dietitian in the state of Texas, and an American Council on Exercise Certified Personal Trainer. A member of the Sports, Cardiovascular, and Wellness Practice Group of the Academy of Nutrition and Dietetics (SCAN), she holds a Doctorate of Philosophy in education and a dual Master of Science Degree in Exercise Science and Human Nutrition.

Jennifer's experience includes almost three years as a US Peace Corps fisheries volunteer in Sierra Leone, West Africa; working in clinical nutrition as a cardiac dietitian; as the chronic-disease nutritionist for a state health department; as a college professor teaching nutrition and sports nutrition; and as a private-practice dietitian providing one-on-one nutrition counseling.

She is the author of seven healthy-eating cookbooks: *The 21-Day Healthy Smoothie Plan*, *Diabetic Cookbook for Two*, *Healthy Smoothie Recipe Book*, *The Alkaline Diet for Beginners*, *The Insulin Resistance Diet for PCOS*, *The Heart Healthy Cookbook for Two*, and *The Complete DASH Diet for Beginners*. Jennifer continues to teach college-level nutrition and sports nutrition, writes, and provides individual nutrition counseling and personal-training services through her online business, Koslo's Nutrition Solutions.

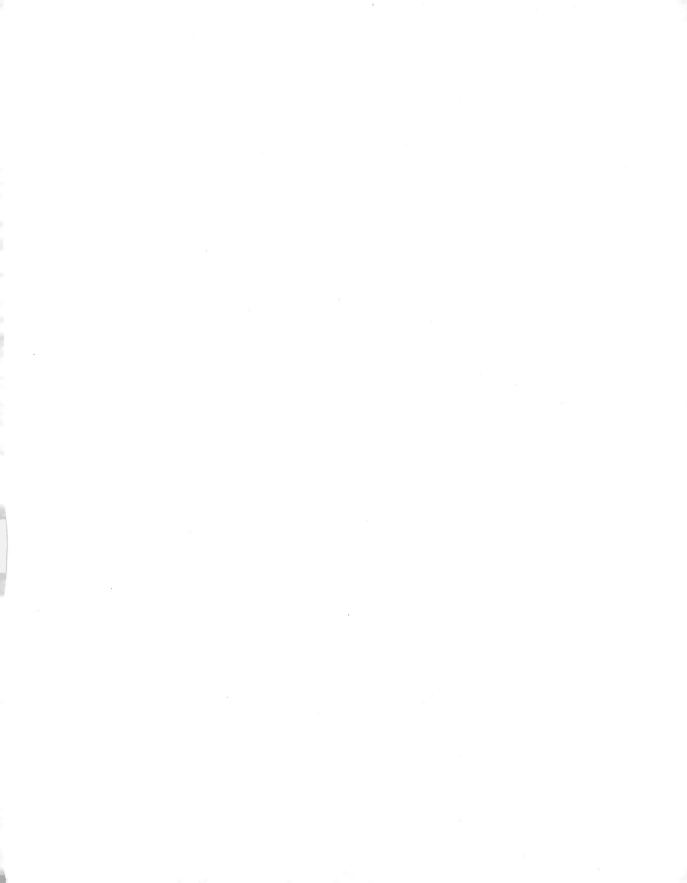

CPSIA information can be obtained
at www.ICGtesting.com
Printed in the USA
JSHW012339010322
23364JS00003BA/6

9 781939 754226